THE BODY SCULPTING BIBLE

EXPRESS

James Villepigue

Hugo Rivera

Photography by:
Peter Field Peck

WOMEN'S EDITION

healthyliving**books**

New York • London

www.bodysculptingbible.com

Published by Hatherleigh Press
5-22 46th Avenue, Suite 200
Long Island City, NY 11101

www.hatherleighpress.com

Villepigue, James C.
 The body sculpting bible express workout for women : featuring the 21-minute express 14-day
body sculpting program / by James Villepigue, Hugo Rivera.
 p. cm.
 Includes bibliographical references.
 ISBN 1-57826-295-3
 1. Bodybuilding for women. 2. Physical fitness for women. I. Rivera, Hugo A., 1974- II. Title.
 GV546.6.W64V54 2004
 613.7'13--dc22
 2004021944

Disclaimer
All forms of exercise pose some inherent risks. The information in this book is meant to
supplement, not replace, proper exercise training. Before practicing the exercises in this book, be
sure that your equipment is well-maintained. Do not take risks beyond your level of
experience, training, and fitness. The exercise and dietary programs in this book are not
intended as a substitute for any exercise routine or treatment or dietary regimen that may have
been prescribed by your doctor. As with all exercise and dietary programs, you should get your
doctor's approval before beginning. The author, editors, and publisher advise readers to take full
responsibility for their safety and know their limits.

THE BODY SCULPTING BIBLE EXPRESS WORKOUT books are available for bulk purchase, special promotions, and premiums. For information on reselling and special purchase
opportunities, please call us at 1-800-528-2550 and ask for the Special Sales Manager.

Special thanks to Marie-Annick Courtier, RoseMarie Alfieri, Lisa Low, and Isabel Zschabran.

Cover design by Deborah Miller
Interior by Deborah Miller and Calvin Lyte

10 9 8 7 6 5 4 3 2 1
Printed in United States

Dedication

I would like to dedicate this exciting project to the most important people in my life. To my remarkable mom, Nancy, I am truly blessed by God to be your son and I simply adore you; to my talented sister, Debbie, my love for you could never cease and I am, as I have always said, "So very proud of you!"; to my awesome dad, Jim, I love you always and I miss you so much, pal. I honor you every moment of my life. To God, thank you, thank you, thank you! To Heather, thank you for your incredible support, I love you; to all of my beautiful family and friends, you know who you are and I love you all! Finally, to those of you reading, thank you so much. We hope you enjoy *Express For Women*. Good luck and God bless!

Additionally, I would like to thank the following people: Andrew Flach and Kevin Moran, you have both become dear friends; a heartfelt thank you for all of the wonderful opportunities you have given me. Thank you, Paul Frediani, you are a class act man! To my bro, Peter Field Peck, as always, great work! To RoseMarie Alfieri, you are so awesome! To all of the Hatherleigh Press team, you are all the very best!

James Villepigue

Dedication

This book is dedicated to my beautiful wife Lina, who always loves and supports me unconditionally throughout any project; to my son Chad, who is my pride and joy; to my parents and grandparents for always believing in me and who always ensured that I would get the best education possible as I grew up; to my brother Raul whose computer knowledge made it possible for me to go online; to my in-laws who are always there to help me and provide me with support in time of need; to William Kemp for being such an awesome mentor and friend; to Chris Lind for all his website help and friendship; and finally to God for giving me the talent to put this work together.

Additionally, special thanks go out to Tim Gardner and Todd Mendelsohn. Without your help, I would not be at the level of development that I am today. Thank you so much for your expertise and your great friendship!   Andre Hudson, for being such an inspirational success story, an awesome trainer, and a great friend. Laree Draper, for always being there to offer a hand and for the incredible job you do maintaining Irononline, the best weight training email group in the Internet. Dave Draper, for always leading by example and for being an inspiration to all who follow the body sculpting lifestyle. The people at Prolab Inc., for giving me the opportunity to get more involved in the fitness industry and for putting out such awesome high quality products at a great price. To RoseMarie Alfieri, for your valuable input and awesome help. Last but not least, Andrew Flach and Kevin Moran. Thank you for giving me the opportunity to spread the fitness word to millions of people.

Hugo A. Rivera

Table of Contents

Precautions

You should always consult a physician before starting any weight gain or fat reduction training/nutrition program.

A basic metabolic test, thyroid, lipid, and testosterone panel is recommended prior to starting this program in order to detect anything that can prevent you from making the most out of your efforts.

Consult your doctor regarding these tests.

If you are unfamiliar with any of the exercises, consult an experienced trainer to instruct you on the proper form and execution of the unfamiliar exercise. Improper form can lead to injury.

The instructions and advice presented herein are not intended as a substitute for medical or other personal professional counseling.

HR Fitness Inc., the editors, and the authors disclaim any liability or loss in connection with the use of this system, its programs, and advice herein.

Introduction
Is This Workout for You?

"I have so much free time I don't know what to do with it!" Have you ever heard anyone you know say this—and actually mean it? Chances are the opposite is true. You're more accustomed to hearing and thinking: "How on earth am I going to do everything I need to do? There's just not enough time." Not enough time to get work done, to enjoy ourselves, to be with our friends and our families. Certainly not enough time to exercise!

That's why the *Body Sculpting Bible EXPRESS* workout—a workout you can do in 21 minutes—was created. This is a workout so efficient, it was designed specifically to help you achieve the greatest fitness gains in the least amount of time possible. You may not have enough time to commit to hour-long workouts at a gym a few days a week. But surely you can spare 21 minutes three or four days each week.

THE **BODY SCULPTING BIBLE** EXPRESS

We all know by now how important it is to incorporate exercise into our lives. Study after study shows that people who exercise are healthier and that physical activity helps to improve our outlook on life. Many of us simply want to look better—to have bodies that are toned and slim. In other words, you must find the time to work out.

THE *EXPRESS* PROGRAM

Maybe you are an extremely busy woman whose calendar reads like your pre-holiday shopping list; perhaps you are a mother of young children, who devotes most of your time and energy to them, but who wants to get back in shape; or maybe you are someone who simply does not want to spend your evenings working out, even if you have the time, or maybe you want to get in and get out, and onto other things you enjoy in life. The 21-Minute *EXPRESS* Workout is for you.

Can you really only work out for 21 minutes and get results? Absolutely. It's a little bit like cooking. There are very complicated, multi-ingredient recipes that take over an hour to prepare and which are delicious. But there are also plenty of quick recipes that use fewer ingredients, take less than a half-hour to prepare, and are still delicious and nutritious. Often we hear people say that they don't feel that it's even worth it to go to the gym if they can't do a long, drawn-out workout. Some people will spend hours at the gym in a very inefficient way (resting too long between exercises, talking away half their workout, performing too many repetitions, or using weight

that is way too light). While they may be at the gym for an hour plus, they are in fact only benefiting from a fraction of that hour. The essential factor in any workout is a proper structure that efficiently puts research exercise science to work for you.

We've designed a three-day-a-week program that covers all of the major muscles in your body: upper body, lower body, and midsection (core)—with a special focus on the legs. We also provide optional abdominal and cardio programs for the other days. In the 21-Minute Workout, you move quickly from one exercise to the other, which enables your heart rate to rise into a training zone to get cardiovascular as well as strength and muscle building benefits. We spell out every step of the workout, so that you know what to do, how to do it, and in what order.

You can use the Body Sculpting Bible *EXPRESS* Workout in a number of ways. It can be your main workout, or it can complement longer workouts or cardio workouts such as running and biking. You can make this the workout you do on those days or weeks when you are pressed for time. It's a great workout to do when traveling as you just need a couple sets of weights. And, it's wonderfully suited for women who are just beginning an exercise program, and want to get good results quickly.

THE 21-DAY CHALLENGE

You will be successful in sculpting your body and enhancing your health and fitness if you make the commitment. In just 21 days, you'll see changes in your body, in the way that you feel, and even the way you think.

That is our challenge to you. Spend 21 minutes a day for 21 days with us, and commit to a higher level of fitness. If you are looking for a jumpstart back into an old routine, this can get you started. If you are looking for a quick set of exercises to keep you fit for life, this is it.

If you're ready to feel stronger, and to know that you are investing in your health and fitness, it's time to take the 21-Day Challenge. At the end, there's nothing that will make you feel better than to look back on your accomplishments.

HOW TO USE THIS BOOK

This book begins with a discussion of the principles of the *EXPRESS* Workout—how and why it works. You'll see that while the workout is short on time, it is long on intensity and this makes all the difference. You'll learn the supporting evidence for this type of workout. We will also present a general protocol for strength training, discussing how to properly lift weights to maximize benefits and minimize risk of injury, and how to set workout goals.

In Chapter 2, we present a general eating plan that supports healthy, active living. You really are what you eat, and you need to make the food choices that will give you the most nutritional bang for the caloric buck. This is especially true when you are exercising and need your body to be full of energy!

Part II presents the exercises that are in the 21-Minute Workout programs. In Chapter 3, we go over the importance of warming up and stretching—a vital, often overlooked, component of any fitness program. You'll find challenging, effective exercises for your back and chest, shoulders and arms, abs, legs, and glutes, as well as a section on combination exercises, which work the lower and upper body at the same time. We've also given you alternative exercises you can do on stack machines if you prefer.

Finally, Part III contains the 21-Day Challenge and your six-week, 21-Minute Workout program featuring workouts that you can perform with just a pair of dumbbells and a bench or step. Optional workouts are included for stack machines at the gym. While machine workouts are good, you'll get the most out of dumbbell workouts. We will explain this in the next chapter.

SUCCESS DEFINED

In the *Body Sculpting Bible,* we talked about what success is. It's worth reiterating here: success depends on desire, determination, and action. You must want to be successful, and want it strongly. You must be determined to overcome any obstacles you may have (often when it comes to exercise, these are psychological) and, finally, you must actually get up and engage in exercise. You must act. If you have these three qualities, the workouts in this book will help you to obtain a sleeker, leaner body. This can be done in just 21 minutes a session— barely any time at all.

Part I

The Principles of the *EXPRESS* Workout

This part will introduce you to the principle of periodization, a method of training that is scientifically proven to give you the best results. We will also give you all the tools you need to maximize your benefits and minimize your risks, including protocols on the proper way to lift weights, meal plans to support your fitness goals, and tips on how to maintain your motivation.

Chapter 1
21 Minutes to Fitness

THE 21-MINUTE SOLUTION; HOW AND WHY IT WORKS

The Body Sculpting Bible *EXPRESS* Workout was created to provide an efficient workout for those of you who do not have more than 30 minutes a day free to dedicate to fitness. For example, we spoke to many school teachers who have a lot of time during the summer, but when school starts, their workout time gets drastically reduced. This is for people like them.

Now, the question is raised: "Is 21 minutes enough time to get results?" The answer is an emphatic yes! We have to remember that, unlike most things in life, working out more and more reaches a point of diminishing returns. Many times, people who are overly enthusiastic

THE BODY SCULPTING BIBLE EXPRESS

1

and who exercise too much begin storing body fat and losing muscle. The reason for this is a stress hormone released by the adrenal glands called cortisol. This hormone is affected by exercise, and while its release can be minimized if workouts are kept short, it is released in large quantities when you work out excessively. When it comes to fitness there is only one thing that you need to remember: intensity. If you focus and work hard during the time you are able to work out, you will accomplish more than the people who spend two hours in the gym talking most of the time.

While the workouts from the original *Body Sculpting Bibles* will provide more rapid results, the *EXPRESS* Workouts will provide comparable results in even less time at the gym. In other words, what you could accomplish during six weeks of using the longer workouts, you will be able to accomplish within roughly 10 weeks of using the shorter workouts. Not bad considering that the time invested is minimal.

SUPPORTING SCIENTIFIC EVIDENCE

A study performed in 2002 by researchers from the University of Minnesota and the Mayo Clinic showed that two short 30 minute sessions a week in the gym is all that adults need to experience effective body fat loss and valuable gains in muscle strength and lean muscle mass (*International Journal of Obesity* 27:326-332, 2002). Sixty women ranging from ages 30 to 50 years old lost an average of two pounds of fat and gained an average of two pounds of muscle in 15 weeks. There was no monitoring of the participants' diets during the study, so we can assume that there was little or no change of eating habits. Also, the workout routine the participants used may not have been as effective as it could have been.

By using the three periodized 21-Minute Workouts described in this book, coupled with the fat-burning, muscle-building diet presented in Chapter 2, you will lose body fat and gain muscle at the fastest rate possible. It is quality, not quantity, that counts the most in the world of fitness.

GOAL SETTING AND THE 21-DAY CHALLENGE

Without goals we are a ship adrift in the middle of the sea. We go with the flow and if we ever get anywhere it is by mere accident. In order to achieve success, we need to clearly define and ingrain our goals in our minds. Otherwise, like the drifting boat, if we get anywhere it will be by mere chance.

This book's goals are designed around the 21-Day Challenge. If you can exercise for 21 minutes a day, every day, for 21 days, you will be well on your way towards getting fit! This workout can be used if you're just beginning and need a starting program for your fitness regime, or if you're returning to the gym after a long absence. This workout lasts for only three weeks, obviously a short-term goal. It's up to you where you want your body to be in the long term.

Do you want to bodybuild, lose inches, or increase your endurance? Decide now, before you even lift a weight. As a small exercise, take out a piece of paper and write down two things. The first will be your long-term goals. Be specific! Write the measurements that you will have (Chest, Arms, Thighs, Calves, and Waist), your body fat percentage and your total body weight. Don't limit yourself to what you think you can achieve; write down what you want. (At the same time, if you are a woman who wants to have a 22-inch waist but whose height is 5'10", this may be an unrealistic goal. Shoot for a 26-inch waist instead.) Did you write down your long-term goals? If not, stop reading and do so now!

If you are reading this paragraph we will assume that you wrote down your long-term goals. Now, the problem is that such goals seem so far away. Since every long trip starts with the first step, write down your short-term goals. For the purposes of this *EXPRESS* Workout, the first three weeks will be jump-starting your fitness regime. It's the second three weeks which will determine your eventual path. Short-term goals should be analyzed every six weeks. Obviously, your short-term goals will be smaller than long-term goals. By having more and more short-term goals, your long-term goals are achievable. When you write down your goals, be positive and have no doubt in your mind that you can achieve them. This is crucial! So go ahead and write your short-term goals down now. Here's the format:

For the next six weeks I will:

Lose	_____	pounds of fat
Gain	_____	pounds of muscle
Weigh	_____	pounds

Have measurements of:

Chest	_____	inches
Arms	_____	inches
Thighs	_____	inches
Calves	_____	inches
Waist	_____	inches

Once you have all of those goals written down, write down what ACTIONS will you take for the next six weeks to get there. For instance:

ACTION PLAN

- I will carry healthy snacks with me to eat between balanced meals

- I will wake up and do cardio first thing in the morning three times a week

- I will do three 21-minute weight-training sessions a week

- I will get a full night of sleep

- I will drink one gallon of water a day

- I will only have one cheat day a week

You can also take pictures of how you currently look (be sure to also document current measurements: body weight, body fat, etc.). This is a great way to stay motivated—when you look at your current pictures, and compare them with pictures of yourself a year later, you will see a huge difference!

Now that you have written all of this down, it is time to move from words to actions. If you follow your action plan religiously and you only miss your goals by a bit, don't get discouraged! You should see progress and this is what we are shooting for; constant progress that will lead us to our ultimate goals.

If you missed your mark because you did not follow your action plan, don't punish yourself. Simply set new goals and be more determined to follow your action plan.

If you mess up your plan for a day, don't drop the whole thing and quit! If you encounter one of these days, begin your recovery the following day by starting the plan again.

Now that you have your goals, we'll talk about the formula for success. After that, we'll present you with an exercise workout that works so that you can go ahead and achieve your plan; the 21-Minute Body Sculpting Bible *EXPRESS* Workout.

THE FORMULA FOR SUCCESS

No matter what your goals are, the formula for success will guarantee that you get the results you want. The only thing that differs is the way in which each individual implements it, because each individual has different goals. For example,

most women like to tone up their waist, legs, and arms while most men are interested in getting large amounts of muscle size everywhere.

The formula is the following:

$$S = D \times (T+N+R)$$

S is the success that you achieve in your program, **D** is the determination that you have to achieve success, **T** is the training that you use, **N** is your nutritional program and **R** stands for rest.

Each component in the formula can be assigned a 0 or a 1. A 1 is given to a component if it is followed completely, and a 0 is given to any component not completed or halfway followed. If every single component is followed, you can get a maximum value of 3. This person will get the fastest results possible from their program. If the person stops training, resting, or eating properly, she will get a smaller value and less than optimal results. However, if you don't have determination, your value is 0 and you won't get any results. Determination is by far the most important factor in your success with your exercise program.

It is now easy to see why purchasing a sophisticated gadget or a couple of magic pills at the health food store is not going to cut it. To achieve permanent results, all of the factors have to be present and in harmony. Follow one but not the other and your success will be negatively affected. Now that you have an idea of what it will take to get the body of your dreams, let's go into each of the individual components of the formula for success.

DETERMINATION

This is the most important by far. If you are not determined enough to make the sacrifices necessary to get in shape, then it's not going to happen. Take the case of one of us (Hugo): *Most people usually think that I have all the time in the world to work out (by the way, most people's excuse for not being in shape is lack of time). When I tell them that I am married, I have a child, and work full time on my business (around 50-60 hours per week) they can't believe it. I can certainly understand that we live in a very busy age. However, please don't tell me that you don't have at least 21 minutes 3 times a week that you can spare to take care of yourself; that is simply unbelievable.* Be determined and stick to your goal!

TRAINING

There are two types of training:

ANAEROBIC WORK (i.e. weight training) is the #1 way to sculpt your body. Why? Weight training is far superior to any other type of exercise because it increases your metabolism, which in turn helps you burn fat, and gives shape to your body.

AEROBIC WORK (i.e. walking) in your Fat Burning Zone (you can calculate your fat burning heart rate with the following formula: (220 – your age) x 0.75) is a good way to accelerate the fat-burning process. You should not overdo it, and this should be used only in addition to a good weight-training program. Aerobics should never be used as a substitute for weight training.

NUTRITION

Nutrition and training go hand-in-hand. Have you ever heard people say that as long as you work out you can eat anything you want because the workout will burn it off? That is wrong! You cannot go every day to McDonald's and get a Big Mac with fries.

If you follow the wrong diet, or follow no eating plan at all, rest assured that your training efforts will be sabotaged and you will have no results at all.

REST AND RECOVERY

You need seven to nine hours of sleep each night for your body to run efficiently. Deprive your body of sleep and your fat loss will suffer. You'll also lose muscle, which in turn will lower your metabolism. You'll also deprive your hormonal production, which makes it difficult to build muscle. Finally, there is research that points to the fact that sleep deprivation may be linked to the following:

1. Heart disease
2. Depression
3. Bad temper
4. Lack of concentration and lethargy
5. Increased risk of breast cancer (Richard Stevens, a cancer researcher at the University of Connecticut Health Center, has speculated that there might be a connection between breast cancer and hormone cycles disrupted by late night light. Melatonin, primarily secreted at night, may trigger a reduction in the body's production of estrogen. However light

interferes with melatonin release (secreted normally in response to a lack of light), allowing estrogen levels to rise. Too much estrogen is known to promote the growth of breast cancers.)

Make sure that you get your ZZZ's or else your body will not be operating at peak efficiency.

STRUCTURE AND PRINCIPLES OF THE WORKOUT: WHY AND HOW IT WORKS

The workout allows for three days of weights and three days of abdominals. The abdominal workout can be done in the comfort of your home at any time and will take you approximately six minutes or so to complete. For faster fat-burning results, an optional vigorous 15-minute cardiovascular session following the abdominals can be performed.

The weight workout splits the body in the following manner:

DAY 1: Full Body Routine using conventional weight training exercises

DAY 2: Problem Area Specialization: shoulders, triceps, thighs, hamstrings, calves

DAY 3: Full Body Routine using combination exercises

This split emphasizes a balanced physique because all major muscle groups are stimulated and also places an emphasis on women's problem spots like legs, shoulders, and triceps.

The *EXPRESS* Workout uses free weights (dumbbells) and the 14-Day Body Sculpting Principles to create the fastest results. The program is based on your body's physiology. It usually takes your body 14 days to get used to a new practice, whether that practice is following a diet, a new exercise program, or just getting up earlier in the morning. Getting used to a new practice, such as waking up early to exercise, is a great thing. However, getting used to an exercise program is not as great. Why? Once your body gets used to it, it will stop responding and your results (i.e. fat loss and increased muscle tone) will come to a screeching halt. That is why most people who go to the gym experience great results initially, but later see and feel themselves going nowhere. The key to experiencing continued results is variation. However, the variation cannot be haphazard. You must have a plan that will guarantee continual results; such as the Body Sculpting Bible *EXPRESS* Workout.

For the first two weeks you will use modified compound supersets. This means performing one exercise, resting a prescribed amount of time, going to the next exercise, resting the prescribed amount of time, and going to the next until the circuit is done. Once the circuit is completed, you start at the beginning and repeat

MONDAY	TUESDAY	WEDNESDAY	THURSDAY	FRIDAY	SATURDAY	SUNDAY
Day 1	Abs/Cardio	Day 2	Abs/Cardio	Day 3	Abs/Cardio	Off
Day 2	Abs/Cardio	Day 1	Abs/Cardio	Day 3	Abs/Cardio	Off

for the recommended amount of times. During this two-week period of modified superset use, your body gets stronger as rest periods are abundant and repetitions are at a higher range (12-15). Working out this way allows your nervous system to recover and your body to increase its strength. In addition, the high repetitions allow your body to build more capillaries (necessary for the delivery of nutrients to the muscle cell) and prepare the joints for the heavier weights to come. On weeks 3 and 4 you will start supersetting, or performing one exercise after the other without rest for some of the exercises. The workout becomes more intense in nature, thus creating a higher demand on the central nervous system. Heavier weights and fewer reps (10-12) with a slightly higher number of sets are used as well. The increased volume and the shock to the body created by the increased stress of the weight training routine causes an increased output of growth hormone (that greatly enhances fat loss and muscle tone) and an increase in your metabolism. When your body adapts to this routine, you further add to the intensity by increasing the number of sets, using heavier weights (8-10 reps) and Giant Sets performing four exercises, one after the other, without rest. Once again the body is shocked, growth hormone output goes through the roof, and your metabolism is jolted. The routine is so intense that if you were to maintain it for more than two weeks you would enter a state of overtraining (a state where your body cannot recover from the demands imposed by the intense routine). When your body reaches this level, you will give your body a

chance to recover for the next couple of weeks by returning to Week 1.

Are you going backwards? Not at all! With this program you are always moving forward. Even though you are going back to a less stressful type of training with less volume, you will notice that you are now stronger on the same exercises that you had previously worked with. You will use greater weights for the 12-15 repetition range because your body naturally built up its nervous system energies to the highest level possible. Now that your exercise is less stressful you'll have all of this extra energy to get even stronger and more muscular. That is how your strength will increase. After two weeks of modified compound supersets, once again you'll begin to increase the stress on your body and continue this results-producing cycle.

Why is it necessary to get strong and why should you lift heavier weights? Building up your strength through progressive resistance training is the key to increased muscle tone and accelerated fat loss. Remember, if your strength stays the same, your body will look the same. And don't worry, these weights will not make you bulky. Women lack the testosterone necessary to achieve huge gains in muscle mass. The women that you may see on professional bodybuilding shows have trained very hard and use very heavy weights to achieve their look. In addition, they use bulk-up diets and many even take anabolic steroids to compensate for their lack of testosterone. Rest assured, you cannot end up looking like a professional female bodybuilder by accident—it takes a ton of hard work and a lot of food!

BEGINNERS AND THE *EXPRESS* WORKOUT

The Body Sculpting Bible *EXPRESS* Workout is designed for women who have at least six weeks of training experience. If you are a beginner, you will need to perform the same routine laid out in the first two weeks of the program for a period of six weeks. It will take your body approximately six weeks to adjust to the movements, and makes this most efficient for recruiting muscle fibers. It will also give your cardiovascular system a chance to get into shape. By the end of the six weeks, you should have lost a significant amount of weight and you should start seeing more muscle tone and definition in your body. You should also be able to reach your target heart rate by the end of this period. Beginners can also jump start their fitness program by taking the 21-Day Challenge presented in Chapter 9.

BEST TIME TO WORK OUT

We recommend you work out in the morning as soon as you awake. Drink 16 ounces of cold water before you start the workout and an additional 30 to 60 ounces during the activity. This is essential to prevent dehydration. We recommend working out first thing in the morning on an empty stomach because you will burn 300 percent more body fat this way. In the morning, your body doesn't have any carbohydrates to burn. In the absence of carbohydrates, your body goes straight to the fat stores in order to get the energy necessary to do the work. Another good reason to work out in the morning is growth hormone levels are at their highest levels (one of the hormones responsible for muscle growth and influencing fat loss).

Working out in the morning will allow you to expedite fat loss for dramatic results. However, we do understand that certain obstacles, such as work constraints, might not permit you to train in the morning. In this case, do your cardio or weight training two or three hours after any meal (if your last meal was at 3 p.m., then your exercise session should be at 5 or 6 p.m.).

WORKOUT CLOTHING

Wear comfortable clothes that allow your body to move freely without constraints. Therefore, rigid clothes like jeans and the like are definitely out of the question. You also need to choose clothes based on the climate and environmental conditions. You should wear extra layers of clothing if it is cold to help keep your body temperature warm and prevent possible injuries. Wear comfortable cross training shoes along with a thick absorbent pair of socks. Never train in your bare feet or with sandals; you could seriously injure your feet if you dropped a plate or a dumbbell.

HOW FAST SHOULD YOU LIFT THE WEIGHT?

This fascinating topic is one that many people in the fitness industry have had difficulty agreeing upon. "Should I lift the weight fast? Should I lift the weight slow? Should I move the weight fast or slow on the positive (concentric) portion of the rep? Should I move fast or slow on the negative (eccentric) portion of the rep?" All of these are very good questions and should all be researched. In fact, we have done the research and will now answer each one in detail.

We have found that slow lifting is usually only good for beginners that have never lifted a weight before. It helps them to learn and master the movement and prevents them from using bad exercise form. However, as you become more advanced, science and our own experience indicate that you should lift the weight as quickly as possible without sacrificing form and without involving momentum (jerking and bouncing of the weights). You create more force lifting fast and therefore more muscle fibers are activated. If you do not use momentum to help move the weight, then the force you generate during the movement is created solely by your muscles and not inertia. This is what helps stimulate your muscles to grow, and creates the tone and shape that you so desire. While some might believe that super slow lifting is beneficial because it is difficult to perform and painful, it is not the best way to stimulate muscle growth. Super-slow lifting accumulates too much lactic acid within your muscles and fatigues them before they reach real momentary muscular failure.

Science tells us that Force = Mass (in this case the weight you are lifting) times Acceleration (the increasing speed at which you lift the weight). Therefore, the best way to lift weights is to lift them fast, with total control of the weight and void of momentum. Since you won't be jerking the weights or using ballistic movements during exercise, the risk of getting injured is no greater than the risk of getting injured lifting super slowly.

One last thing about lifting speed: If you are lifting a weight that only allows you to do 8 repetitions, it might look like you are lifting the weight slowly even though you are lifting it as fast as possible. This is due to the fact that the heavier the weight the slower you will be able to move it, even though you are trying to accelerate as fast as you can. This is amazing! We are sure you've heard people's concerns about how lifting heavier weights is dangerous, right? It is actually the opposite. When you lift lighter weights, you have the ability to move the weights very quickly and sloppily because little stress is put upon the muscles, tissues, and joints. This creates a greater risk for injuries to occur. When you lift heavier weights, you are forced to go slower and to use controlled form. Lifting heavier weights will stimulate more muscle fibers while limiting the chance for injury. On the other hand, do not lift a weight if you cannot lift it for a minimum of eight repetitions. Heavier weights may indeed cause connective tissue injury.

HOW TO BREATHE WHILE PERFORMING THE EXERCISE

The correct way to breathe while performing an exercise is to exhale (breathe out) while you are forcing the weight up (the concentric phase a.k.a. muscle contraction) and to inhale (breathe in) while you are lowering or releasing the weight (the eccentric phase a.k.a. the negative portion of the exercise). For example, if you are doing a bench press, you exhale while you push the weight away from your body and inhale while you lower the weight towards your chest.

MUSCLE SORENESS

Muscle soreness is caused by microtrauma to the muscles and is a good indicator that the workout you performed was effective. If you have never exercised before, you will experience higher levels of soreness than usual at the beginning of your program. That is OK. As your body gets used to the exercise program, the muscle soreness will subside to tolerable levels. You just need to persevere through those first few weeks. Do not confuse this type of soreness with overtraining.

There are several degrees of soreness that you need to be aware of:

- Delayed Onset Muscle Soreness
- Typical Mild Muscle Soreness
- Injury-Type Muscle Soreness

The first type of soreness is delayed onset muscle soreness (DOMS). The term DOMS refers to the deep muscular soreness usually experienced two days (not the day after) after the exercise has been done. DOMS prevents the total muscular contraction from occurring within a muscle. This type of severe soreness is caused when you either embark on an exercise program for the first time or when you train a body part harder than usual. It can last for a couple of days for an advanced well-conditioned athlete or for as long as a week for a beginner. If this type of soreness is affecting you and it is time to work out again, the best thing to do is to exercise the affected body part in an active recovery routine. In active recovery routines, all of the loads are reduced by 50 percent, and the sets are not taken to muscular failure. For example, if you are to perform an exercise for 10 repetitions, divide the weight that you

usually use for that exercise by two. Stop performing the exercise even though you may not reach muscular failure at the tenth rep. Active recovery helps to restore full movement in the muscle, helping to remove the lactic acid and other waste products building up within the muscles. It also forces high concentrations of blood into the damaged area of the muscles and nourishes the muscles for repair and growth. We find that doing this is always beneficial; by the next day you will not be as sore or stiff as you ordinarily would have been had you skipped a workout to wait for the pain to subside.

The second type of soreness is the typical mild muscle soreness experienced the day after a good workout. While scientists are still unable to pinpoint the true cause of such soreness, the explanation generally accepted is that it is caused by microtrauma at the muscle fiber level and by an excess of lactic acid. At any rate, what's important is that this is a good mild soreness that does not impair muscle function like DOMS. The pain generally lasts a day for advanced athletes and up to three days for a beginner. This soreness, on average, indicates that you had a good workout the day before because you created the trauma necessary to trigger adaptation (e.g. muscle growth). When you are no longer experiencing this type of soreness, it is a good indication that your body has successfully adapted to the training program. This is not one of the goals you will be striving for, as it leads to no gains. And, this is the reason why our program changes on a consistent basis.

The third type of soreness is the one caused by injury. This soreness is entirely different in nature from the ones described above, as it is usually immobilizing and triggers very sharp pain within the muscles and/or joints. Depending on the nature of the injury, the pain might either be experienced constantly or only when the joints are moved or muscles contract. These injuries often become apparent as soon as they happen. Other times they appear either the day after and sometimes days after the activity. If you suddenly become injured, the first thing that you should do is apply the RICE principle (Rest, Ice, Compression, and Elevation). After consulting a doctor, who might allow you to continue training, carefully work around the injury (in other words, utilize exercises that work around the injured muscle(s), without overstepping the range of motion that triggers the pain). More serious injuries, such as a muscle tear, may involve complete rest of the injured and surrounding areas and, depending on the severity, possibly surgery. The best way to prevent this type of injury, pain, and soreness, is by cycling your exercise parameters and by constantly practicing good form.

OVERTRAINING

Overtraining is a condition caused when the body is taxed beyond its ability to recover. The main causes may include long workouts, an overload of training volume (too many sets and reps), a poor diet, lack of sleep, etc. People experiencing this condition might notice such symptoms as a loss of muscle mass, weakness, trouble sleeping, loss of appetite, a lethargic and constant tired feeling, or feelings of depression.

It is impossible to overtrain with our weight-training program (assuming you follow the nutrition and rest practices) because after you stress the body's recuperative capabilities to the maximum (by doing supersets for two weeks and then moving on to Giant Sets for two more), you back off into the less stressful modified compound supersets. In addition, you get a rest day after every day of lifting and the weekends off. During rest days, you concentrate on optional fat burning aerobic exercise (that aids in the recuperation process by removing the lactic acid created by weight training). Sunday is our total inactivity day. This day serves to rest the body and the mind. Finally, the short duration of the workout coupled with ample nutrients provided by the diet, along with the recommended supplements, eliminate the possibility of getting overtrained.

Provided that you follow the training program as laid out, in conjunction with the nutrition and rest components, you should not suffer from overtraining.

HOW TO SELECT THE WEIGHT FOR EACH EXERCISE

The weight you select for each exercise depends on the number of repetitions that you need to do for a particular set. If you need to do between 10-12 repetitions for one set, then you need to pick a weight where you fail (the point at which completing another repetition becomes impossible) between 10-12 reps. This takes a bit of practice but after a while you will become extremely accurate when it comes to choosing the correct weight for a particular repetition range. If you pick a weight that allows you to do more than 12 repetitions, you'll need to increase the amount of weight being lifted. If you reach failure before hitting the 10th rep, you'll need to decrease the amount of weight. For example, if you are doing four sets of an exercise, as you work through the sets, fatigue will set in and you may not be able to continue using the weight that you chose to lift during the first set. When you get to the point where you can no longer lift a particular weight for a pre-determined repetition range, simply decrease the weight and prepare yourself for the next set.

MISSING WORKOUTS

Missing workouts is unacceptable. You hear it all the time: people making excuses about having no time to exercise. Unless you are on call 24 hours a day, you can find the time to train. If you are interested in completely changing the way you look and feel, all the excuses in the world cannot hold you back from doing what it takes to fit a workout into your schedule. All you need is the vision, the motivation, and the determination to do so.

Missing workouts will severely jeopardize your toning and fat-burning efforts, and destroy your bodysculpter's mindset. If for some reason you are not able to train then make up the missed session the next day. This might mean sacrificing your Sunday rest day or weight-training on abs/optional cardio day, in which case you can either do both workouts at the same time (extending the length of the session to around 45 minutes) or have several sessions that day.

In conclusion, if you miss a workout for whatever reason, don't beat yourself up. Tomorrow is a new day and you will be able to make up the missed session. However, don't make a habit of missing training sessions, as missing sessions will ultimately limit your results.

EQUIPMENT NEEDED

The workout routines in this book use dumbbell-based exercises. Training must consist primarily of free weight exercises in order to bring about the fastest results because these exercises recruit the most muscle. In addition, the body is designed to be in a three-dimensional universe. Whenever you use a machine, you limit your body to a two-dimensional universe and consequently limit the number of muscle fibers doing work.

Not all machines are bad. Some definitely have a place in our weight-training program because they isolate the muscle in a way that no free weights can. However, our program should be based on dumbbell exercises for the reason explained above and also because this fast moving routine is performable at home or at a crowded gym just by getting some dumbbells and a bench. (You can use a step instead of a bench if you prefer.)

MACHINE-BASED ROUTINES FOR VACATION

Typically hotels do a good job of having weight machines in their fitness rooms but lack free weights. Because of this, the book includes a machine-only routine that you can use when on vacation. All you have to do is use the routine corresponding to the week that you were on in order to keep from missing workouts. For instance, if you were on weeks 3-4 of the free weights program, use the machine-based routines presented under those same weeks. While you do not get as much benefit as you would from a free weight routine, you can still continue your workouts, which is far better than not working out at all.

Chapter 2
Eating for Health and Fitness

In order to make impressive changes in your figure, nutrition and training need to go hand in hand. It is a myth that a person can eat as much as they want as long as they exercise. Only people with extremely fast metabolic rates (rate at which the body burns calories) can get away with this. Having said that, with so many diets on the market, we understand why it can be difficult to know what sort of nutrition program is best to follow for the fastest results.

Before covering the diet that we feel is most appropriate based on our personal experiences and clients' results, we'll cover some nutrition basics.

THE BODY SCULPTING BIBLE EXPRESS

2

NUTRITION BASICS

There are three macronutrients that the human body needs in order to function properly.

CARBOHYDRATES

Carbohydrates are your body's main source of energy. When you ingest carbohydrates your pancreas releases a hormone called insulin. Insulin is very important because:

1. It grabs the carbohydrates and either stores them in the muscle or stores them as fat.

2. It grabs the amino acids (protein) and shelters them inside the muscle cell for recovery and repair.

Most overweight people on low fat/high carbohydrate diets eat too many carbohydrates, releasing too much insulin and thus storing fat. There are complex carbohydrates and simple carbohydrates. The complex carbohydrates give you sustained energy ("timed release") while the simple carbohydrates give you immediate energy. You should eat mainly complex carbohydrates throughout the day except for your post-workout meal.

STARCHY COMPLEX CARBOHYDRATES: oatmeal, sweet potatoes, potatoes, rice, grits, or cream of rice.

FIBROUS COMPLEX CARBOHYDRATES: broccoli, carrots, cauliflower, green beans, lettuce, mushrooms, pepper, spinach, or zucchini.

SIMPLE CARBOHYDRATES: apples, bananas, grapefruit, grapes, oranges, pears, pineapple, or peaches.

PROTEIN

Proteins are the building blocks of muscle tissue. Without it, building muscle and burning fat efficiently would be impossible. It increases your metabolism every time you eat it by up to 20 percent, and helps with carbohydrates' timed release.

Everybody involved in a weight-training program should consume between 1 to 1.5 grams of protein per pound of lean body mass (meaning that if you are 100 pounds, and have 10 percent body fat, you should consume at least 90 grams of protein since your lean body mass equals 90 pounds). Nobody should consume more than 1.5 grams per pound of lean body mass as this is unnecessary and the extra protein may get turned into fat.

Good examples of protein are eggs, chicken breast, turkey, 90% lean red meats, and tuna.

FATS

All the cells in your body have some fat in them. Hormones are manufactured from fats. Fats also lubricate your joints. If you eliminate the fat from your diet, your hormonal production will plummet and a whole array of chemical reactions will be interrupted. Your body will then start accumulating more body fat than usual so that it has enough fat to keep on functioning. Since testosterone production is halted, so is muscle building. Therefore, in order to have an efficient metabolism we need fat.

There are three types of fats: saturated, polyunsaturated, and monounsaturated.

SATURATED FATS: Saturated fats are associated with heart disease and high cholesterol levels. They are found to a large extent in products of animal origin. Some vegetable fats also contain large amounts of saturated fats and are generally found in packaged foods. Coconut oil, palm oil, palm kernel oil, and non-dairy creamers are also highly saturated.

POLYUNSATURATED FATS: These fats do not have an effect in cholesterol levels. Most of the fats in vegetable oils, such as canola oil, corn oil, cottonseed, safflower, soybean, and sunflower oil are polyunsaturated. When you consume this fat, it should be from flaxseed oil and fish oils. They are usually high in the essential fatty acids and may have antioxidant properties.

MONOUNSATURATED FATS: These fats have a positive effect on the good cholesterol levels by lowering the bad and increasing the good cholesterol. Sources of these fats are extra virgin olive oil and nuts such as cashews, pecans, and almonds. Peanuts fit in here too although it is really a bean rather than a nut. The main source of your monounsaturated fats should be extra virgin olive oil.

We recommend that 20 percent of your calories come from good fats. Any less than 20% and your hormonal production decreases. Any more than 20% and you start accumulating plenty of fat. Good sources of fat are extra virgin olive oil, natural peanut butter, flaxseed oil, and fish oils.

THE LOW-CARB MYTH

Today the dieting craze is low-carb dieting, where carbohydrates are reduced to 30-50 grams per day in an effort to accelerate weight loss.

So, do these diets work? They do in a way, but not any better than what we call the balanced approach. The key to ensure that the low-carb diets work is to take most of the allotted carbohydrates in the form of vegetables like broccoli and green beans. Your saturated fats are limited to no more than 30 grams per day and most of your fat intake comes from extra virgin olive oil, fish oils, and flaxseed oil. Nuts are good too but they have carbohydrates so you have to be careful with them.

I (Hugo) have used these types of diets for as long as a year with the modifications described above and here are my conclusions:

If you are only allowed 30-50 grams of carbohydrates a day, your life will not be very tasty. You will only be limited to a small selection of foods.

Even though at the beginning you lose incredible amounts of weight, it is mostly water weight. I also did not find a big difference between losing fat in a low-carb diet versus fat on a moderate carbohydrate diet like the one described in the following section.

While on a low-carbohydrate diet, the muscles feel flat (shrink in size) because glycogen (carbohydrates stored inside the muscle cell that make the muscles look firm) is depleted.

DRINK WATER

Water is by far the most abundant substance in our body. Without water, an organism would not survive very long.

- Over 65 percent of your body is composed of water (most of the muscle cell is water).

- Water cleanses your body of toxins and pollutants.

- Water is needed for all of the complex chemical reactions your body performs on a daily basis, such as energy production, muscle building, and fat burning. A lack of water interrupts all of these processes.

- Water helps lubricate the joints.

- When the outside temperature rises, water serves as a coolant to bring the body temperature down.

- Water helps control your appetite. Sometimes when you feel hungry after a good meal this sensation indicates a lack of water. Drinking water at that time would take the craving away.

- Cold water increases your metabolism.

In order to know how much water your body needs a day, just multiply your lean body weight by 0.66. The resulting number indicates how many ounces of water you need in a day.

On a moderate carbohydrate diet, your muscles always feel firm and tight.

I experienced joint pains after the ninth month. I was drinking two gallons of water a day, so lack of fluids was not the problem. Once I switched back to a moderate carb diet, the joint pains disappeared.

You have to pay close attention to your cholesterol levels and to nutritional deficiencies caused by the lack of variety in the diet. In order to get all the good fats in the diet, I had to take them in liquid form—not very tasty.

Even though this diet might work, it will be hard to maintain for a lifetime. As a matter of fact, we see that most people are so restricted on this plan that once they go off, they become compulsive overeaters. While this does not happen to everyone, it does happen. Also, after a few months on the diet, your weight loss plateaus as your thyroid adjusts downward due to the lack of carbohydrates. This in turn lowers your metabolism.

If you feel like trying a low-carb diet, please remember to pay close attention to your cholesterol levels and nutritional deficiencies. Finally, keep in mind that while you can eat slightly more calories on a low-carb plan without storing them as fat, there is a caloric limit after which you will start storing body fat even in the absence of carbs. Therefore, like any diet, remember to create a small caloric deficit.

Having said all this, we believe that to get in shape the best approach is a more balanced diet like the one in the following section.

THE BALANCED APPROACH

In the balanced approach, we use a diet that contains all of the macronutrients in a balanced manner. The breakdown of the nutrient ratios for your diet looks like this:

40% Carbs
40% Protein
20% Fats

CHARACTERISTICS OF A GOOD NUTRITION PROGRAM

YOUR NUTRITION PLAN SHOULD BE BASED ON EATING SMALL AND FREQUENT MEALS THROUGHOUT THE DAY.

When you feed your body several times a day, your metabolism greatly increases. Your body uses food as energy to fuel your metabolism efficiently, burning more fat. If you neglect to feed your body, and wait over three or four hours for consumption, your body switches to a catabolic state and believes it is starving. It begins to feed on your lean muscle tissue, your body's water, your organ tissue, and begins to store your ingested calories as fat for future use. The diet industry has made us think that the key to losing fat is an extreme restriction of calories, but this is not true!

During the Body Sculpting Bible *EXPRESS* program, try to eat between five to six meals a day.

YOUR MEALS SHOULD CONTAIN CARBOHYDRATES, PROTEIN, AND FAT IN THE CORRECT RATIOS.

When you eat a meal that does not contain the proper balance of nutrients (for example, an all carbohydrate meal such as pasta), you will not yield the desired results. Every macronutrient has to be present in order for the body to absorb and use them efficiently. If you only eat carbohydrates, your energy levels will drop in about 30 minutes and unused carbs will be stored as body fat. If you eat only protein, your energy will be low and your body cannot turn protein into lean muscle tissue. The ratios for each particular macronutrient have to be correct to get the results that you desire.

NO SMOKING AND LIMITED ALCOHOL CONSUMPTION.

Both lower testosterone levels (among many other potential problems). Alcohol in particular is greatly responsible for increased fat gain since each gram of alcohol has 7 calories, mostly derived from carbohydrates.

CALORIC REQUIREMENTS

Caloric requirements for most women fluctuate between 1200 and 1500 calories per day. However, if you eat the same number of calories day in and day out, your body will get used to that amount and you will stop losing fat. Therefore, we recommend that you alternate between 1200 and 1500 calories. For two weeks you will consume 1200 calories, and then the following two weeks you will consume 1500.

Once you know the total number of calories you need to take in every day, calculate the amount (in grams) of each nutrient by using the percentages below:

Total amount of carbs for the day = (Total number of calories x 0.40)/4

Total amount of protein for the day = (Total number of calories x 0.40)/4

Total amount of fat for the day = (Total number of calories x 0.20)/9

Note: Carbs and protein are divided by four because there are four calories per gram of carbs or of protein. For fats, we divide by nine since there are nine calories for every gram of fat.

Dividing all of the results from the formulas above by five (by six if you are eating six times a day) gives you the amount of each nutrient that you will need to consume per meal. As you see, you will be eating between five and six times a day to keep your metabolism high. You don't have to ensure that you get the exact amount that the formula gives you at each and every meal, however, make sure that you stay within +/-10 grams of the formula when counting protein and carbs and +/-5 grams when counting fats.

CHOOSING WHAT TO EAT

One of the biggest challenges we face when starting a diet is deciding what to eat every day. Now that you have calculated the amount of carbs, protein, and fats you need for each meal, you need to choose what foods to eat. For this purpose, the food groups table found in Appendix B contains the food values

---

1500-CALORIE WEEK MACRONUTRIENT REQUIREMENTS

150 grams of carbohydrates (mostly complex, with simple carbs being saved for after the workout)

150 grams of protein

33 grams of fats

In six meals that comes out to approximately:

25 grams of carbs per meal

25 grams of protein per meal

6 grams of fats per meal

---

for the foods we recommend you eat should you wish to alter the sample meal plan on the following pages. It is very accurate. However, with so much food processing going on in the food industry these days, it can get tricky. If you happen to discover a discrepancy between the nutritional information on a food label and the chart, believe the food label instead, as we cannot tell what additives they might have decided to add to their ingredients.

Change the times in the Sample Meal Plan to fit your own schedule (we have used the typical 8 a.m.-5 p.m. work day). The post-workout meal assumes that you are training in the morning. If this is not the case, then just have some complex carbs in the morning and move the post-workout meal to the time after your workout is done.

SAMPLE MENU

On the following pages, we have given you a

complete menu plan that will aid you in constructing your diet. Remember to have lower calories for two weeks and higher for the following two! If you would like to adapt this menu to your own schedule and liking, please see Appendix B for instructions and food charts.

STRIVE FOR CONSISTENCY INSTEAD OF ABSOLUTE PERFECTION

Many times we see dieters that start out doing great. However, there comes a day that for some reason they miss a workout or they blow their diets. After that day, they become so discouraged that they continue missing workouts or destroy their diets with self-sabotage. Many weeks go by before they get back on track (if ever). In the meantime, muscle tone fades and fat pounds pile up. Please remember the following: we are all human and we are entitled to make mistakes. Always strive for perfection, but if for some reason things don't go as well as they should on a given day, pick up and move on.

1200-CALORIE WEEK MACRONUTRIENT REQUIREMENTS

120 grams of carbohydrates (mostly complex, with simple carbs being saved for after the workout)
120 grams of protein
26 grams of fats

In five meals that comes out to approximately:

24 grams of carbs per meal
24 grams of protein per meal
5 grams of fats per meal

Jump right back into your program. If you blow a meal one day, don't make it any worse by eating incorrectly all day long. If you miss a workout, don't wait until next Monday to start over. Just continue with your program the way it is laid out. In the end it will be your determination and consistency that will enable you to win the battle of the bulge.

TROUBLESHOOTING YOUR CALORIC INTAKE

The optimum fat loss per week is two pounds. Any more than two pounds a week and you will lose muscle, which will result in the loss of muscle tone, which yields a saggy look and a significantly lower metabolism. Having said that, we need to point out the fact that while most women burn between 1200 to 1500 calories, some have a higher metabolism. Therefore, some women may find themselves losing more than 2 pounds a week at the prescribed number of calories and others may find themselves gaining weight. If this is the case, don't panic! If you find you are losing too much, simply add 300 calories to both the lower calorie diet and the higher calorie diet. In this manner, your diet will fluctuate between 1500 and 1800 calories. After two weeks you should assess how this is working by measuring your lean body mass. If you are still losing weight after two weeks, again increase calories by an additional 300 and repeat the process until you reach the caloric intake that allows for a 2-pound fat loss while at the same time adds muscle tone.

The reverse applies if you are suddenly gaining weight. If you are gaining, cut your calories

MENU PLAN FOR LOW CALORIE WEEKS (2 Week Duration)

Meal 1   (7:30 AM)

CARB OPTIONS:
- 1/2 cup of dry oats mixed with water   -or-
- 3 tablespoons of Farina (measured dry)   -or-
- 3 tablespoons of cream of rice (measured dry)   -or-
- 1/2 cup of grits (measured dry)

SIMPLE CARBS (assuming this is a post workout meal; otherwise switch this with the meal that falls after your workout):
- 1 medium banana

PROTEIN OPTIONS:
- 1/2 cup of Egg Beaters (measured uncooked)   -or-
- 1 scoop of whey protein (approximately 20-25 grams of protein)

Meal 2   (10:30 AM)

PROTEIN SHAKE:
- Meal replacement shake such as Prolab's Naturally Lean Matrix   -or-
- 1/2 scoop of protein powder such as Prolab's Protein Component mixed with 8 ounces of skim milk

GOOD FATS:
- 1 teaspoon of flaxseed oil

Meal 3   (12:30 PM)

CARB OPTIONS:
- 1/2 cup of brown or white rice   -or-
- small sized baked potato   -or-
- small sized sweet potato   -or-
- 1/2 cup of oatmeal (measured dry)

VEGETABLE OPTIONS (Fibrous Carbs):
- 1 cup of green beans mixed with any other desired vegetable   -or-
- 1 cup of broccoli mixed with any other desired vegetable

PROTEIN OPTIONS:
- 3 ounces of chicken   -or-
- 3 ounces of turkey   -or-
- 3 ounces of lean fish such as tuna, grouper, red snapper   -or-
- 3 ounces of 97% lean steak such as top round sirloin

Meal 4   (3:30 PM)

PROTEIN SHAKE:
- Meal replacement shake such as Prolab's Naturally Lean Matrix -or-
- 1/2 scoop of protein powder such as Prolab's Protein Component mixed with 8 ounces of skim milk

GOOD FATS:
- 1 teaspoon of flaxseed oil

Meal 5   (6:30 PM)

CARB OPTIONS:
- 1/2 cup of brown or white rice   -or-
- small sized baked potato   -or-
- small sized sweet potato   -or-
- 1/2 cup of oatmeal (measured dry)

VEGETABLE OPTIONS (FIBROUS CARBS):
- 1 cup of green beans mixed with any other desired vegetable   -or-
- 1 cup of broccoli mixed with any other desired vegetable

PROTEIN OPTIONS:
- 3 ounces of chicken   -or-
- 3 ounces of turkey   -or-
- 3 ounces of lean fish such as tuna, grouper, red snapper   -or-
- 3 ounces of 97% lean steak such as top round sirloin

Meal 6   (8:30 PM)

CARB OPTIONS:
- You may choose any of the carb options from Meal 1 or 3 but for if fat loss is the main goal then limit carbs to the fibrous choices below:

VEGETABLE OPTIONS (FIBROUS CARBS):
- 1 cup of green beans mixed with any other desired vegetable   -or-
- 1 cup of broccoli mixed with any other desired vegetable

PROTEIN OPTIONS:
- 3 ounces of chicken   -or-
- 3 ounces of turkey   -or-
- 3 ounces of lean fish such as tuna, grouper, red snapper   -or-
- 3 ounces of 97% lean steak such as top round sirloin   -or-
- 1 scoop of protein powder such as Prolab's Protein Component mixed with water

GOOD FATS:
- 1 teaspoon of olive oil

RECOMMENDED SUPPLEMENTS:

MULTIPLE VITAMIN/ MINERAL PAKS:
PROLAB's Training Paks

MEAL REPLACEMENT POWDERS:
PROLAB's Naturally Lean Matrix

PROTEIN POWDERS:
PROLAB's Protein Component

FLAXSEED OIL:
Spectrum's flaxseed oil as it is always kept refrigerated on the way to the retail store.

If following the Advanced Program, the following supplements may also be useful:

CREATINE:
PROLAB's Creatine Monohydrate Powder

GLUTAMINE:
PROLAB's Glutamine Powder

MENU PLAN FOR HIGH CALORIE WEEKS (2 Week Duration)

Meal 1 (7:30 AM)

CARB OPTIONS:
3/4 cup of dry oats mixed with water   -or-
4 tablespoons of Farina (measured dry)   -or-
4 tablespoons of cream of rice (measured dry)   -or-
3/4 cup of grits (measured dry)

SIMPLE CARBS (assuming this is a post workout meal; otherwise switch this with the meal that falls after your workout):
1 large banana

PROTEIN OPTIONS:
3/4 cup of Egg Beaters (measured uncooked) -or-
1 scoop of whey protein (approximately 20-25 grams of protein)

Meal 2 (10:30 AM)

PROTEIN SHAKE:
Meal replacement shake such as Prolab's Naturally Lean Matrix -or-
1/2 scoop of protein powder such as Prolab's Protein Component mixed with 8 ounces of skim milk

GOOD FATS:
1 teaspoon of flaxseed oil

Meal 3 (12:30 PM)

CARB OPTIONS:
3/4 cup of brown or white rice   -or-
medium sized baked potato   -or-
medium sized sweet potato   -or-
3/4 cup of oatmeal (measured dry)

VEGETABLE OPTIONS (Fibrous Carbs):
1 cup of green beans mixed with any other desired vegetable -or-
1 cup of broccoli mixed with any other desired vegetable

PROTEIN OPTIONS:
4 ounces of chicken   -or-
4 ounces of turkey   -or-
4 ounces of lean fish such as tuna, grouper, red snapper   -or-
4 ounces of 97% lean steak such as top round sirloin

Meal 4 (3:30 PM)

PROTEIN SHAKE:
Meal replacement shake such as Prolab's Naturally Lean Matrix   -or-
1/2 scoop of protein powder such as Prolab's Protein Component mixed with 8 ounces of skim milk

GOOD FATS:
1 teaspoon of flaxseed oil

Meal 5 (6:30 PM)

CARB OPTIONS:
3/4 cup of brown or white rice   -or-
medium sized baked potato   -or-
medium sized sweet potato   -or-
3/4 cup of oatmeal (measured dry)

VEGETABLE OPTIONS (Fibrous Carbs):
1 cup of green beans mixed with any other desired vegetable   -or-
1 cup of broccoli mixed with any other desired vegetable

PROTEIN OPTIONS:
4 ounces of chicken   -or-
4 ounces of turkey   -or-
4 ounces of lean fish such as tuna, grouper, red snapper   -or-
ounces of 97% lean steak such as top round sirloin

Meal 6 (8:30 PM)

CARB OPTIONS:
You may choose any of the carb options from Meal 1 or 3 but for if fat loss is the main goal then limit carbs to the fibrous choices below:

VEGETABLE OPTIONS (Fibrous Carbs):
1 cup of green beans mixed with any other desired vegetable -or-
1 cup of broccoli mixed with any other desired vegetable

PROTEIN OPTIONS:
4 ounces of chicken   -or-
4 ounces of turkey   -or-
4 ounces of lean fish such as tuna, grouper, red snapper   -or-
4 ounces of 97% lean steak such as top round sirloin   -or-
1-1/2 scoop of protein powder such as Prolab's Protein Component mixed with water

GOOD FATS:

RECOMMENDED SUPPLEMENTS:

MULTIPLE VITAMIN/ MINERAL PAKS:
PROLAB's Training Paks

MEAL REPLACEMENT POWDERS:
PROLAB's Naturally Lean Matrix

PROTEIN POWDERS:
PROLAB's Protein Component

FLAXSEED OIL:
Spectrum's flaxseed oil as it is always kept refrigerated on the way to the retail store.

If following the Advanced Program, the following supplements may also be useful:

CREATINE:
PROLAB's Creatine Monohydrate Powder

GLUTAMINE:
PROLAB's Glutamine Powder

BEVERAGE TIPS

Many dieters can literally just blow their diets without realizing that they're doing it. The culprit? Drinking the wrong types of beverages.

Drink plenty of water daily. Your recommended fluid intake should be 0.66 x body weight in ounces per day.

Absolutely no regular sodas or fruit juices, even the ones that claim to be all natural. They contain too many simple carbs. For example, the average soda contains 40 grams of sugar while an 8-ounce serving of the average fruit juice contains between 25-35 grams of simple carbs!

Crystal Lite beverages and decaffeinated tea/coffee are OK as long as they are used in moderation; your main beverage should be water.

Try to avoid alcohol. An occasional glass of red wine is OK provided that you are of legal drinking age.

by 150 for both the lower calorie diet and the higher calorie diet. You'll notice that we did not cut the calories by quite as much, as your metabolism might only need a 150-calorie deficit. If you find that you are still gaining, even after the 150 calorie cut, you may than decrease your calories by the additional 150 calories. Don't jump the gun! Give your body the opportunity to adjust.

EATING ON THE RUN: FAST FOODS

Today's hustle and bustle can really tax your abilities to plan and prepare. This preparation certainly includes the scheduling of food consumption. If, for one reason or another, your time constraints don't allow you to prepare all of the food you need for the day, or if you run out of food, there is a solution. You can go to a fast food restaurant. But aren't fast foods bad if you are trying to get in shape? The answer is no—as long as you choose wisely.

The rules for eating in fast food restaurants (or any other type of restaurant) are set below:

- If it is not your cheat day (see the Sunday Reward) refrain from fatty choices such as french fries.
- Drink between 8-16 ounces of water before you get to the restaurant and then drink an additional 8-16 ounces while you eat. This will prevent you from feeling hungry and falling to temptation. If you find that temptation is strong remember two things:
  (1) There is nothing better than being in shape.
  (2) You control everything that goes into your mouth. Food does not and should not control you!
- Always combine a serving of low-fat protein (in the case of fast food restaurants, this is either skinless chicken or turkey) with a small serving of carbs. Remember that if you are eating a chicken or turkey sandwich, the bread will count as the carbs.
- Salads in addition to a serving of protein and a serving of starchy carbs are always good since they provide fiber and fill you up. However, avoid using high fat/high sugar dressings.

• Refrain from using high carbohydrate sauces or mayonnaise.

Now that we know the rules of fast food eating, see the box below for some healthy meals you can choose at some of the major fast food chains.

If you find yourself in another restaurant we haven't discussed, don't panic! Just ask for a chicken plate and if it comes with skin, just take it off. Basically, if you stick to the five rules dis-cussed above, no matter where you find yourself, you won't have a problem finding something to eat. Bon Appetit!

THE SUNDAY REWARD

For one meal each Sunday we want you to cheat on your diet. You can go to a restaurant, have a nice appetizer, a main meal and a dessert. Much more cheating than this (having two appetizers and three desserts, for instance) and you risk

---

FAST FOOD CHOICES

In **Arby's** you can have either a Light Chicken Deluxe Sandwich with extra lettuce and tomato (no mayo) or a Light Turkey Deluxe Sandwich. They also have an excellent roast chicken salad that will not harm you unless you fill it up with high fat dressing.

In **Bennigan's** try the chicken platter, which includes a serving of spicy rice along with vegetables and two chicken breasts.

In **Boston Market** for protein you can have a serving of turkey breast or chicken breast. For carbs, you can have a small serving of steamed vegetables along with potatoes, or corn, or rice pilaf or fruit salad. If you'd rather have something quicker, then go for the chicken or turkey sandwich.

In the **Golden Corral** try the chicken (remove the skin) with their steamed rice and green beans.

In **Hardee's** order either a chicken fillet sand-wich or grilled chicken salad.

In **Kentucky Fried Chicken** have a quarter chicken (no skin) for protein and a small serving of mashed potatoes, or garden rice, or red beans for carbs.

In **Long John Silver's** you may have a flavor-baked chicken or fish for protein and a small serving of plain baked potato or green beans.

In **McDonald's** you can have either a McGrilled Chicken Classic or a Chunky Chicken Salad.

In **Subway** order a Roast Turkey Breast Sub, a Veggie Sub or a Roast Beef Sub. Remember the rules that we already discussed: no extra oils or mayo etc. Also, there is no need to order a sub larger than 6 inches.

In **Taco Bell** order any of the following: a Light Chicken Burrito, or a Light Chicken Taco, or a Light Bean Burrito, or a Light Soft Taco Supreme, or a Light Taco Supreme, or a Light Taco, or a Light Soft Taco.

Finally, in **Wendy's** have either a grilled chicken sandwich or a grilled chicken salad.

going backwards. You can only reward yourself in this way if you have stayed on track the rest of the week. One cheat meal a week is actually beneficial since it confuses your body and increases your metabolism. By cheating, you prevent your body from adjusting to the diet, which can lower your metabolism. It also removes the psychological fear that you will never be able to eat bad foods again. Having said that, we must caution that some people (us included) find it hard to go back to good dieting if they incorporate cheat foods in their diets once a week. They fall into a non-stop binging with these foods that may last for weeks. Do not feel bad if you fall into this category. Like we said, we are in this boat as well. It is natural to crave foods that are bad, considering that they taste so darn good. If you fall into this category and feel tempted or need to still build your willpower, stick to a healthy diet and stay away from cheat meals until you have reached a confident level of empowerment.

THE IMPORTANCE OF PREPARING FOOD BEFOREHAND

Preparation is crucial to the success of your dietary program. If you are not prepared, you will fail! Life is too hectic to eat five or six times a day without a little bit of preparation.

One thing you can do is to prepare your food the night before and store it in individual containers that have a section for complex or simple carbs, a place for fibrous carbs, and a place for protein. You also can prepare protein shakes the night before and store them individually in containers purchasable at the grocery store. When the following day comes, all you have to do is take out the container that has breakfast, heat it up, and eat. Then

COOKING TIPS

Follow the guidelines below to ensure proper food preparation:

- Eat vegetables raw or slightly steamed. If boiling, be careful not to overcook or you will lose the nutritional value of the vegetables.

- Do not fry. Always broil, grill, steam, or bake (broiling, grilling, and steaming are better as they allow fat to drain while cooking).

- Trim all fat from meat and remove skin from poultry prior to cooking.

- Do not use salts, butter, oils, or sugar while cooking. Experiment with herbs, non-salt seasonings, lemon juice, vinegar, garlic, and pepper, even a touch (1 tbsp, not a bottle) of some white or red wine. Occasional use of salsa, low sodium soy sauce, catsup, and mustard to enhance meats and vegetables is OK if used sparingly (1 tbsp). Minced white or green onions are also excellent for seasoning.

grab the container for lunch and two protein shakes, put them in the cooler and go to work. Take a water bottle everywhere you go so you do not dehydrate while at work. When you come home, take out the container for dinner, re-heat it, eat it, and prepare the food for the following day.

If you think you will be able to stick to the plan without being prepared, you place yourself at risk. You will either end up eating the wrong kinds of food, or missing meals. You will definitely spend more money, because eating out is not cheap. Therefore, remember to be prepared!

MEAL FREQUENCY AND WORK

Choose from among these alternatives to make sure you get your five or six meals in each day:

Have breakfast, lunch, and dinner as real meals and keep the rest of the meals as meal replacement protein shakes. Protein bars are discouraged as recent research indicates that even the low carb bars increase insulin levels by as much as a sugar loaded bar.

Have all of your meals as real meals by convincing your boss to have three 20 minute breaks instead of a full hour lunch so you can eat all of your meals.

In my experience, the more real food you eat the better the results. High-level bodybuilders know this and that is the reason that the last few weeks before a contest they will eat as much as eight real meals per day!

PROTEIN SHAKES

It's better to eat as much real food as possible, but if you are too busy to fix four to six real meals, you can substitute meals with a shake. You can have either a meal replacement packet mixed with water or a scoop of protein mixed in skim milk with a teaspoon of flaxseed oil (refer to the supplements section for more information). However, make sure that you eat at least two real meals a day (three being preferred).

EMOTIONAL EATING

In our fast-paced, high-stress society, many people resort to emotional eating for comfort. This is a dangerous activity; if this happens very often, the weight will begin to pile on. Also dangerous is the fact that emotional eating usually occurs at night after work.

If you feel like you engage in emotional eating, remember the reasons why you embarked in this program on the first place. Also, keep in mind that overeating is not going to solve any problems and will prevent you from getting the results you deserve. Always ask yourself: "Am I eating this because my body needs it or because I need it emotionally?" Stop to think about what is most important for you. Is it the food or your goals? If it's late at night, go to bed and rest assured that the craving will go away by the time the morning comes.

NOTES ON SUPPLEMENTATION

For this program it is advised that the following supplements be used in order to ensure that there are no nutritional deficiencies:

- A good multiple vitamin and mineral formula taken preferably with your post-workout meal or at breakfast on non-workout days to avoid any nutritional deficiencies. Make sure that it has at least 500mg of calcium, or get a separate calcium supplement such as calcium citrate, which is best absorbed by the body.

- Chromium Picolinate (200 mcg) also with the post-workout meal or at breakfast. This mineral is good for increasing acceptance of insulin. A good insulin sensitivity is necessary in order to optimize the fat burning process. Note: Some multiple vitamin/mineral formulas already have this, so check the label.

- 1000 mg of Vitamin C three times a day. Start with only 500mg and increase the dosage by 500mg per week until you reach the 3000mg total. This is in order to avoid any stomach problems. Vitamin C is fantastic at reducing cortisol levels, which is the stress hormone released by the adrenal glands that eats muscle and stores fat.

- Whey Protein Shakes or Meal Replacement Shakes like Prolab's Naturally Lean Matrix, which is based on complex carbohydrates and a blend of different proteins consisting of a 40/40/20 macronutrient ratio. It contains 20 grams of carbs, 20 grams of proteins and 4 grams of good fats making it the perfect meal replacement supplement for this program. The product is also instantized: it requires no blender just some water and a spoon and the taste is fantastic.

Part II

The Exercises

Here are all the exercises you will need to sculpt the body of your dreams. We've given you soothing stretches to warm up and cool down, challenging exercises for every body part, combination exercises for the most efficient workouts, and alternative exercises you can do on stack machines if you prefer.

Chapter 3

Warm Up and Stretch Out

The pre-workout warm up and post-workout stretch are vital components of your Body Sculpting Bible *EXPRESS* Workout. And they don't require a lot of time—just a few minutes. The next few pages will show you how to warm up most effectively for your workout and how to stretch out your muscles to prevent injury.

WARM UP BEFORE YOU WORKOUT

Research indicates that you should perform an active warm up before you begin a workout. The purposes of the warm up are many: to increase blood flow to the muscles you will be working, to increase your heart rate, to increase your body temperature and warm your joints, improving your flexibility, and to prepare your neuro-

THE BODY SCULPTING BIBLE EXPRESS

3

muscular system for the movements you will need to perform.

The best way to warm up for the Body Sculpting *EXPRESS* Workout is to perform about five minutes of a combination of squats, jumping jacks, and jogging or fast walking. In your warm up try to use all of the muscles you will be working during your *EXPRESS* workout, including your arms.

WHEN TO STRETCH

While there's little evidence that static stretching (the type of stretch that involves holding a stretched position for a number of seconds with no bouncing) before your workout prevents injury, you can do a few pre-workout stretches that are dynamic. Dynamic stretches involve performing several repetitions of bringing a muscle quickly into a stretched position and then immediately releasing it. This type of stretching helps to prepare your muscles for the workout ahead.

Recent research strongly indicates that the best and safest time to do static stretching is at the end of the workout. This is when your muscles are warm due to increased blood flow, and therefore it is the best time to elongate them. In addition, there's less risk of overstretching when the muscles are warm. In contrast, if you perform static stretches on cold muscles (for example first thing in the morning), your range of motion is much more limited and you risk pushing the stretch too far and injuring the muscle or connective tissues.

HOW TO PERFORM THE STATIC STRETCH

Begin your static stretch by inhaling from your diaphragm (the base of your lungs) rather than from your chest. A helpful mental image is to imagine you are inflating a balloon with your breath. As you move into the stretch position, exhale. Go deep enough into a stretch to feel tension in the muscles you are stretching. Never force a stretch. Hold the stretch position for 10 to 30 seconds before releasing. Continue to breathe deeply while in the stretch position. As you hold the stretch, you will begin to feel your muscles moving from a state of tension to relaxation. At this point, you can try to take the stretch a bit deeper. It is normal to feel some discomfort during the initial moments of the stress, but if you feel any pain, ease up on the stretch immediately.

YOUR STRETCH PROGRAM

The stretches that appear on the following pages can be done dynamically pre-workout, or statically post-workout. Before you exercise, perform several repetitions of each stretch, holding each one for only 1 to 3 seconds. After your workout, perform one repetition of each stretch but hold without bouncing for as long as 30 seconds.

THE CAT

A yoga favorite, this stretch warms up and stretches the lower back and abdominal muscles.

TECHNIQUE AND FORM

1 Begin on your hands and knees with your back slightly curved.

2 Exhale as you round your back and pull your abdominals up into your spine.

TRAINER'S TIPS

Make sure that your wrists are under your shoulders and your knees are directly under your hips.

UPPER BACK AND BICEPS STRETCH

This terrific stretch is for the muscles in the middle and upper back, and the front of your arms.

TECHNIQUE AND FORM

1 Start in a standing position.

2 Interlock your fingers and exhale as you press your arms forward (palms facing front) pull your abs into your spine, and round your chest.

TRAINER'S TIPS

✪ Keep your knees slightly bent as you perform the stretch.

✪ Your legs should remain still while you stretch. Only your arms and torso move.

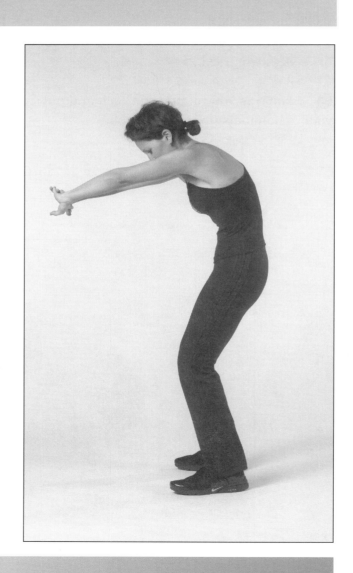

CHEST STRETCH

This is a simple chest stretch that will open up your chest and help to improve your posture. It can be performed either seated or in a standing position.

TECHNIQUE AND FORM

1 Sit cross legged on the floor or mat, or stand with feet placed wide.

2 Bend your arms behind your head, with your elbows facing in front of you.

3 As you exhale, pull your elbows out to the side of your head until you feel a stretch across your chest.

TRAINER'S TIPS

When you pull your arms back, also concentrate on contracting your back muscles. This will intensify the stretch.

STANDING HAMSTRING STRETCH

This stretch relieves tension in the hamstring muscles at the back of your legs. These muscles tend to be tight in most people, so be sure to ease into the stretch position slowly.

TECHNIQUE AND FORM

1 Begin in standing position. Bend from the waist, pulling your abs in to your spine. At the same time extend your left leg, while you bend your right knee.

2 Place your hands on your left thigh and press into the stretch position.

3 Repeat on the other leg.

TRAINER'S TIPS

Try not to lock out your leg as you stretch, and always maintain a slight bend in the knee.

You can make this stretch more intense by varying the position of the leg being stretched. Try placing your leg up on a bench or a chair as you stretch.

SEATED INNER THIGH STRETCH

Many people have limited flexibility in their inner thighs; take care not to overdo this stretch.

TECHNIQUE AND FORM

1 Sit on the floor or mat with your heels pressed together and your knees out to the side. Place your hands around your ankles.

2 As you exhale, press your elbows against your thighs, trying to press your thighs closer to the floor.

TRAINER'S TIPS

Really think about pressing your thighs down against the floor as you execute the stretch.

This is a great stretch to have someone help you out with. Your helper kneels behind you and gently but firmly presses her hands against your thighs, lowering them toward the floor.

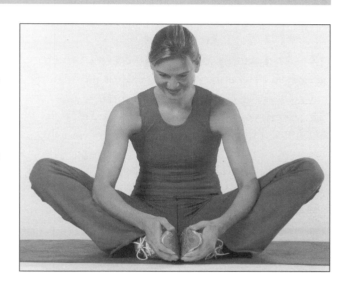

THIGH STRETCH

The classic quadriceps stretch for the front of your thighs can change in intensity depending upon the angle of the stretch.

TECHNIQUE AND FORM

1   Stand, supporting yourself against a wall or by holding onto a pole.

2   Bend your opposite leg behind you, bringing your heel in toward your buttocks.

3   Grasp your foot with your free hand and press in until you feel the stretch in the front of your thigh.

4   Repeat with the other leg.

TRAINER'S TIPS

⊗   Keep your abdominals engaged throughout this stretch.

⊗   To intensify the stretch you can lean a bit forward from the hips.

⊗   Make sure your knee is in line with your hips and not pressed out to the side.

⊗   As an extra balance challenge try this exercise without holding onto the pole or pressing against a wall. If you focus your eyes on a point straight ahead of you, you will increase your ability to balance.

STANDING CALF STRETCH

This stretches the lower muscles in the back of your leg that, when too tight, can cramp up and make you prone to injury.

TECHNIQUE AND FORM

1 Stand straight with your left knee bent about one foot in front of you and your right leg extended a little more than one foot behind your body.

2 Place your hands on your left thigh as you lean slightly forward from the hips, and press your right heel into the floor.

3 Repeat with other leg.

TRAINER'S TIPS

⚙ Breathe deeply into the stretch. Make sure that your heel is in contact with the floor. If you can't touch down, bring your back leg in closer to your body.

⚙ Keep your head in line with your neck by looking straight ahead, and keep your shoulders pulled back and pressed down as you perform this stretch.

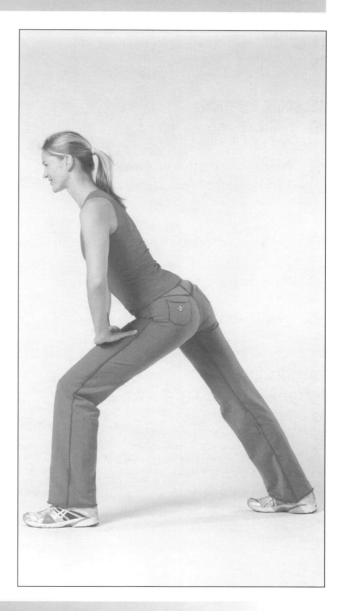

TRICEPS STRETCH

When you perform the triceps stretch for the back of your arms, make sure that you concentrate on reaching your hand down your back as you press your elbow in.

TECHNIQUE AND FORM

1 Stand or sit cross-legged.

2 Reach your right arm straight overhead, then bend it so that your right hand is reaching down your back.

3 Use your left hand to press your right elbow close to your head; at the same time reach down your back with your right hand.

4 Repeat with the other arm.

TRAINER'S TIPS

⊗ Exhale deeply as you reach your hand down your back.

⊗ Make sure your fingers remain unclenched.

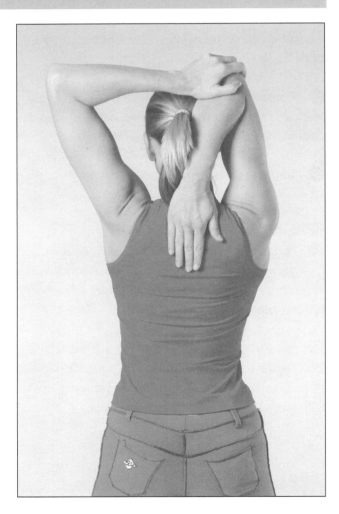

SHOULDER STRETCH

This is an excellent way to stretch the shoulders and thus prevent injury.

TECHNIQUE AND FORM

1 Stand straight. Grasp one of your elbows with the opposite hand.

2 Without moving your torso, pull your arm as far as possible toward your body.

3 Repeat with the other arm.

TRAINER'S TIPS

Keep your arm parallel to the floor as you pull it toward your body.

Keep your legs about shoulder width apart for balance and support.

Chapter 4
Back and Chest

This chapter includes exercises for two of your body's large muscle groups—the back and chest. Your back and chest actually contain several muscles and are ideal to train in a time-efficient workout like the *EXPRESS* Workout. When you exercise your back, you train not only the specific back muscles such as the rhomboids, traps, and lats, but you also train the smaller assisting muscles in your arms—the biceps and deltoids. Likewise, when you train your chest, in addition to working the pectoralis major and minor (the chest muscles) you build the helping muscles in the arms: the triceps and the anterior delts. Our back muscles generally tend to be in greater need of toning than our chests. Many women have weak back muscles from days spent hunched over a computer or desk, or from carrying children and packages. Working on your back helps your waist look smaller and improves your posture, giving you that confident, strong appearance.

THE BODY SCULPTING BIBLE EXPRESS

4

ONE-ARM ROW—PALMS FACING TORSO

The one-arm row is a variation of the two-arm bent-over row. It involves less lower back involvement and is particularly suited for people with back problems, or who do not yet have strong enough abdominal and other core muscles to lift two weights in good form. Two machine exercises with similar movements are the Two Arm Row Machine and the Wide Grip Pulldown Machine.

TECHNIQUE AND FORM

1 Place your right knee and right hand on a bench or chair for support.

2 Bend at the waist until your upper body is nearly parallel to the bench or chair.

3 Lean into your right hand to help support your body weight. You will be training the left side of your back.

4 Pick up a weight with your left hand so that your palm faces your torso. Continue to support your back with your right side. This will be your starting position.

5 Lift your left elbow up toward the ceiling as you exhale. Squeeze and hold in the top position for a second.

6 Slowly lower back to the starting position as you inhale.

7 Repeat for desired number of repetitions.

8 Switch sides and perform the same exercise for the right side of your back.

TRAINER'S TIPS

⊗ Be sure to keep your abdominals pulled in tightly as you lift the weight.

⊗ Keep your arm at your side and your head in line with your spine.

⊗ Avoid twisting or turning your torso.

ONE-ARM ROW—PALMS FACING TORSO

INCLINE DUMBBELL BENCH PRESS

The incline dumbbell press targets your upper chest muscles. Performing this exercise with dumbbells requires your stabilizer muscles to work to keep the weights balanced. In addition to dumbbells, you will need a step or bench for this exercise. A similar machine exercise is the Bench Press Machine.

TECHNIQUE AND FORM

1 Sitting on the step or bench with dumbbells on your thighs, thrust one leg up, leveraging one dumbbell up to your chest.

2 Immediately thrust the second dumbbell upward at the same time as you allow momentum and the dumbbells to guide you back into an inclined position. Use your abdominal muscles to ease you into position.

3 Press the weights straight up to the ceiling. Keep your chest lifted, your elbows out and wide, and your forearms perpendicular to the floor.

4 Lower the weights slowly, making sure your body remains in good alignment.

TRAINER'S TIPS

As you perform the exercise, make sure that you pull your shoulder blades back against the bench (this is called retraction). This allows your chest to do more work than your shoulders.

At the top of the movement you have the option of touching the dumbbells together and squeezing your chest or of pressing the weights straight up. As a variation, you can also turn your palms toward each other at the top of the movement.

INCLINE DUMBBELL BENCH PRESS

VARIATION

ONE-ARM ROW—PALMS FACING REAR

The one-arm row is a variation of the two-arm bent-over row. It involves less lower-back involvement and is particularly suited for people with back problems, or who do not yet have strong enough abdominal and other core muscles to lift two weights in good form. There are two machine exercises that may be substituted for this: the Two Arm Row Machine and the Wide Grip Pulldown Machine.

TECHNIQUE AND FORM

1 Place your left knee and left hand on a bench or chair for support.

2 Bend at the waist until your upper body is parallel to the bench.

3 Lean into your left hand to help support your body weight. You will be training the right side of your back.

4 Pick up a weight with your right hand so that your palm faces to the rear. Continue to support your back with your right side. This will be your starting position.

5 Lift your right elbow up toward the ceiling as you exhale. Squeeze and hold in the top position for a second.

6 Slowly lower back to the starting position as you inhale.

7 Repeat for desired number of repetitions.

8 Switch sides and perform the same exercise for the left side of your back.

TRAINER'S TIPS

Be sure to keep your abdominals pulled in tight as you lift the weight.

Keep your arm right next to your side, your head in line with your spine, and look straight ahead throughout the exercise.

Avoid twisting or turning your torso.

ONE-ARM ROW—PALMS FACING REAR

FLAT DUMBBELL BENCH PRESS

This exercise focuses on the muscles in the middle of your chest. Use either a step or a bench for this exercise. For a similar machine exercise, try the Bench Press Machine.

TECHNIQUE AND FORM

1 Sitting on the step or bench with dumbbells on your thighs, thrust one leg up, leveraging one dumbbell up to your chest.

2 Immediately thrust the second dumbbell upward at the same time as you allow momentum and the dumbbells to guide you back into a lying position. Use your abdominal muscles to ease you into position.

3 Keep your back flat by pulling your abdominals in.

4 Beginning from a position where your elbows are slightly lower than the bench, press the weights straight up toward the ceiling, keeping your chest lifted, your elbows out and wide, and your forearms parallel to the floor.

5 Lower the weights slowly, making sure you keep your back pressed into the bench.

TRAINER'S TIPS

As you perform the exercise, make sure that you pull your shoulder blades back against the bench (this is called retraction). This allows your chest to do more work than your shoulders.

At the top of the movement you have the option of touching the dumbbells together and squeezing your chest or of pressing hem straight up. As a variation, you can also turn your palms toward each other at the top of the movement.

Variety is the spice of exercise, so try the exercise different ways to keep your muscles alert and challenged.

Always keep your elbows perpendicular to the floor.

FLAT DUMBBELL BENCH PRESS

ALTERNATIVE

Chapter 5

Shoulders and Arms

The shoulders and arms are probably the most underrated parts of the body—not thought about very often—and yet most women feel particularly feminine and sexy when wearing a shoulder-baring dress or top. Good posture, well-defined shoulders, and sleek shapely arms add grace and sensuality to your body. The exercises on the following pages will help to get the front and back of your arms and shoulders in top shape—and don't worry, they won't bulk you up.

THE BODY SCULPTING BIBLE EXPRESS

5

DUMBBELL UPRIGHT ROWS

This exercise works not only your shoulders, but your upper back as well.

TECHNIQUE AND FORM

1 Stand in a neutral alignment. Your body should be straight, with your head in line with your spine, knees slightly bent and shoulder-width apart, and a natural curve to your lower back. Hold a weight in each hand with your palms facing the front of your thighs.

2 Exhale and lift the dumbbells up toward your chest by bending your elbows. Lift only as high as your chest to avoid hurting your shoulders.

TRAINER'S TIPS

Keep your elbows out and above the weights as you lift.

Pull your shoulder blades back as you lift the dumbbells.

Concentrate on moving your upper arm and squeezing your shoulder and upper back muscles. This will stimulate the shoulder and upper back muscles more effectively.

DUMBBELL UPRIGHT ROWS

BENT-OVER LATERAL RAISES

This is an awesome exercise that targets the back of the shoulders (the rear delts), thus providing a full, muscular, three-dimensional appearance to the shoulder complex. For a similar machine exercise, try the Reverse Fly Machine.

TECHNIQUE AND FORM

1 Stand in a neutral position, then bend over at your hips. Bend your knees, and keep your back straight and lean forward.

2 Lift the dumbbells out to the sides of your body—to shoulder height—keeping your arms slightly bent at the elbows.

3 When you reach the top position, hold it momentarily before returning to the start position.

TRAINER'S TIPS

To help keep your back straight throughout the exercise, pull your abdominals in tight.

BENT-OVER
LATERAL RAISES

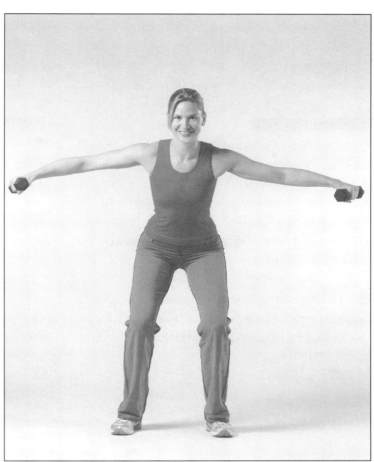

DUMBBELL CURLS

These exercises are for the biceps. You can also perform this with a barbell instead of dumbbells if you want to go heavy on the weights but protect your wrists. There are two equivalent machine exercises: the Biceps Curl Machine and the High Pulley Cable Curls.

TECHNIQUE AND FORM

1 Stand in neutral alignment with your abs held in and a natural curve to your spine. Hold a dumbbell in each hand. Your arms are slightly bent at the elbows and your palms face out.

2 Slowly curl the dumbbells up toward your shoulders, without moving your elbows.

3 Once you reach the top position, hold for a moment contracting your biceps as hard as you can before returning to the starting position.

TRAINER'S TIPS

Be careful not to sway back or forward while executing the curl. If you do, you may be using weight that is too heavy.

Make sure your arms are not locked out when in the down position. This will place too much pressure on your biceps and make you vulnerable to injury.

Perform the biceps curls with a great deal of control, being careful not to use momentum to lift the weights.

DUMBBELL CURLS

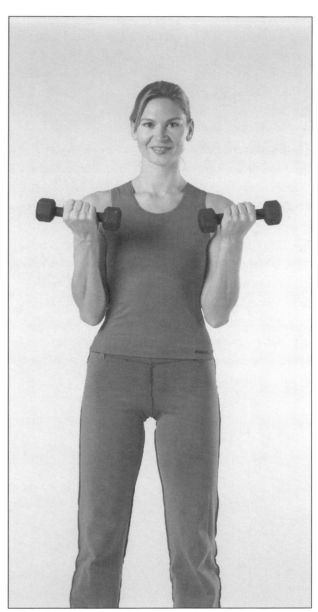

LYING DUMBBELL TRICEPS EXTENSION

The triceps are three muscles located at the back of your upper arm; this exercise focuses on the outer muscles. You can also perform it in a standing position, but lying down is a safer alternative. Two similar machine exercises are the Triceps Pushdown Machine and the Triceps Extension Machine.

TECHNIQUE AND FORM

❶ Lie down on your back, and with a dumbbell in each hand, press your arms toward the ceiling. Your palms should face each other.

❷ Bend your elbows to lower the dumbbells toward your head. The upper part of your arms should remain frozen in place—only your forearms move during this exercise.

❸ Once the weights come close to your forehead slowly press them back up to the starting position (with arms extended).

❹ Hold that position and squeeze your triceps hard.

TRAINER'S TIPS

✪ Concentrate on your form and on accentuating the contraction when you extend your arms; this will more completely stimulate your muscles.

✪ Even though you are straightening your arms over your head, always maintain a slight bend to your elbows for safety.

✪ You can maintain more tension in your triceps by keeping your upper arms slanted in on an angle toward your head.

LYING DUMBBELL TRICEPS EXTENSION

Chapter 6
Abs, Legs, and Glutes

Women love to work their lower bodies. How often do your friends complain about the flabbiness of their abs, glutes, or thighs? It's not an imaginary obsession. The truth is because of their hormonal makeup, women do gain weight in their hips, legs, and abdominals. This is especially true as menopause approaches, when estrogen levels drop along with metabolism. The exercises in this section address the all-important lower body muscles, providing tightening exercises for the legs, butt, thighs, and abdominals. Say goodbye to jumping and inhaling your way into your favorite pair of jeans.

A word of advice: you can work your abs throughout the day by pulling your abdominals in toward your spine when you are sitting, walking, etc. If you are pregnant and in your second or third trimesters, it is advisable not to perform exercises in the supine (laying flat down on your back) position as they can cut off blood supply to your baby. An exercise like a standing crunch is ideal.

THE BODY SCULPTING BIBLE EXPRESS

6

LYING LEG RAISES

This exercise focuses on the lower abdominals and also helps to strengthen the lower back. It must be done properly. If done incorrectly you can hurt your lower back. Focus is essential.

TECHNIQUE AND FORM

1 Lie on your back with your legs extended straight and flat on the floor.

2 Place your hands face down under your buttocks, fingertips facing each other to support your lower back. Also, bend your knees slightly.

3 Lift your legs a few inches off the ground and hold. (Go higher if you need to avoid feeling pain in your lower back.)

4 Squeeze your abs as hard as you can and hold for a couple of seconds.

5 Slowly lower your legs closer to the floor.

TRAINER'S TIPS

Think, think, and think about this exercise as you do it. Focus and feel your abs working as you raise your legs up.

If you feel any pain in your lower back, stop the exercise.

LYING
LEG RAISES

CRUNCHES

Although there are plenty of fancy abdominal exercises around these days, the basic crunch remains one of the most effective for the abs.

TECHNIQUE AND FORM

1   Lay down on your back with your knees bent and your feet on the floor.

2   Cross your hands in front of your chest (beginning) or bend them behind your head (intermediate).

3   Pull your abs in and exhale as you move your chest up toward your knees.

4   At the top position, contract your abs as hard as you can and hold for a couple of seconds.

5   Return to the bottom position, without letting your shoulders touch the floor, and immediately begin the second repetition.

TRAINER'S TIPS

How high you come up is not important. Focus on getting the strongest contraction in your abs.

If you place a folded bath towel under your lower back you can increase the range of motion of the crunch and therefore engage more muscle stimulation.

CRUNCHES

VARIATION

THE BICYCLE

This exercise, commonly known as the bicycle, is very effective when done properly. In a study conducted by the American Council on Exercise, it was found to be one of the most effective exercises you can do to stimulate the muscle fibers in the abdominal area.

TECHNIQUE AND FORM

1 Lie on your back, keeping your hands behind your head and your knees bent.

2 Crunch up as you start, twisting your right side toward your left knee and extending your right leg.

3 Switch sides immediately, brining your right knee in as you extend your left leg.

TRAINER'S TIPS

Try to keep your back pressed against the floor. Avoid having it arch up.

The extended leg should be a few inches off the floor. If you place it too close to the floor you can strain your back.

When you twist toward your knee, actively think about twisting with your waist, rather than with your elbow. If you feel that you are pulling against your neck, you may be using your arms rather than your waist to twist.

THE BICYCLE

THE PLANK

A staple of yoga classes, the plank works the deep internal muscles of your core, including your back. (Maintaining the plank position is also a tough workout for your arms and shoulders.)

TECHNIQUE AND FORM

1 Lie on your stomach, with your forearms against the floor and your legs extended behind you.

2 Lift your body up, keeping your forearms against the floor. Make sure that you keep your back as straight as possible, avoid arching or curving your back.

3 Hold the position for 10 seconds.

4 Lift the right arm and left leg simultaneously and hold for five seconds.

5 Switch sides and hold for five seconds.

6 Relax into the starting position.

TRAINER'S TIPS

⊗ If your core isn't strong enough to maintain a neutral position for your spine, you may lift your hips up a bit until you get stronger.

⊗ Make sure you keep your head in line with your spine throughout this exercise.

THE PLANK

V-KNEE

This very challenging exercise is more advanced; work up to it.

TECHNIQUE AND FORM

1 Sit with your legs straight out in front and your arms bent at the elbows, palms pressed against the floor.

2 Lean back and bring your legs up, balancing on your sit bones. Feel the contraction in your abdominals.

3 Slowly bring your knees in toward your chest at the same time as you lift your chest toward your knees.

TRAINER'S TIPS

To increase the intensity of this exercise you can try performing it with your hands off the floor and out in front of you. You also can add a twist to your torso as you lift. These alternatives should only be performed when you have sufficient core strength to perform the basic exercise.

V-KNEE

VARIATION

LOWER BACK EXTENSION

This exercise, also known as the Cobra or Sphinx, is a great strengthener of the erector spinae muscles in your lower back.

TECHNIQUE AND FORM

1 Lie on your stomach with your legs extended behind you and your hands pressed against the floor.

2 Exhale and lift your torso.

3 Hold that position for a couple of seconds.

TRAINER'S TIPS

Keep your hips in contact with the floor throughout the exercise.

If you feel any pain in your back do not continue this exercise.

If you cannot extend your arms fully, you can keep your forearms on the floor and lift your chest.

LOWER BACK EXTENSION

STAND
AND CRUNCH

Here's one that's a good alternative if you are pregnant.

TECHNIQUE AND FORM

1 Stand in a neutral position, with your back in a slight, natural arch and your arms by your side.

2 Exhale as you pull your abdominals in toward your spine and bend slightly forward. Hold the contraction for a couple of seconds.

3 Straighten to start position.

TRAINER'S TIPS

Really think about this one. Focus on making a deep, strong contraction, as if you are literally squishing your abs against your backbone.

STAND AND CRUNCH

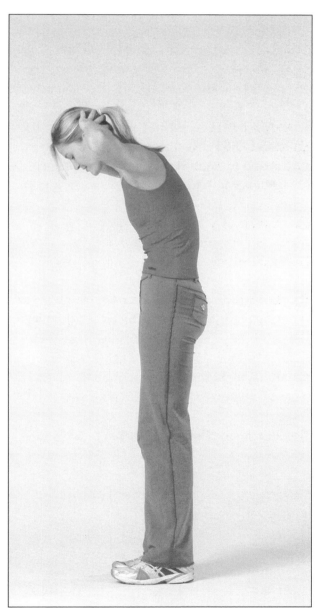

DUMBBELL SQUATS

The squat is one of the most effective and efficient exercises you can do for many of the muscles in the legs, including your glutes, hamstrings, and quadriceps. Not only do squats help develop shapely legs, but they involve recruitment of your core muscles and work balance and stability as well. For a machine equivalent, try the Leg Extension Machine.

TECHNIQUE AND FORM

1 Stand in neutral position, with your feet about hips width apart. Hold a dumbbell in each hand.

2 Bend at your knees and press your hips out behind you.

3 Lower into the squat position (go no lower than the point where your thighs are parallel to the floor—any lower and your risk knee injury).

4 Exhale, pulling your abdominals in, and slowly come up to the standing position.

5 Inhale and lower back down to the squat position.

TRAINER'S TIPS

Keep your body weight centered over your heels rather than your toes, this will help you to be in the right position when you squat down.

Keep your knees in line with your toes.

DUMBBELL SQUATS

STATIC DUMBBELL LUNGES

The lunge also works all the major muscles of your lower body, and is more challenging than the squat for balance. Try the Leg Extension Machine as a machine alternate to this exercise.

TECHNIQUE AND FORM

1 Stand in neutral position, with your legs about shoulder width apart.

2 Step forward with you right leg. Keep your head, shoulders, and hips in alignment.

3 Bend both legs so that your right knee makes a 90-degree angle with the floor and left knee comes close to the floor.

4 Lift up and return to the starting position (as you lift make sure you push off with the right foot).

5 Repeat the desired number of repetitions on the right leg before switching to the left leg.

TRAINER'S TIPS

Concentrate on keeping your back straight throughout the lunge. Avoid leaning forward.

Make sure you bend your back leg so that it almost touches the floor. It is far better to perform this exercise slowly in a full range of motion than to rush through it and come down only half way.

STATIC DUMBBELL LUNGES

WIDE-STANCE DUMBBELL SQUATS

The wide-stance squat is similar to the dumbbell squat, but your legs are wider apart causing greater emphasis on your inner quads and inner thighs.

TECHNIQUE AND FORM

1 Stand in neutral position, with your feet one and a half times wider than your shoulders and your toes pointed to the side. Hold a dumbbell in each hand.

2 Bend at your knees and press your hips out behind you.

3 Inhale as you lower into the squat position (coming no lower than the point where your thighs are parallel to the floor. Any lower and you risk knee injury).

4 Exhale, pull your abdominals in and slowly come up to the standing position.

5 Inhale and lower back down to the squat position.

TRAINER'S TIPS

Be careful not too take too wide of a stance, as this may injure your inner thighs or knees.

Keep your back straight and your head up in line with your spine throughout the squat.

WIDE-STANCE DUMBBELL SQUATS

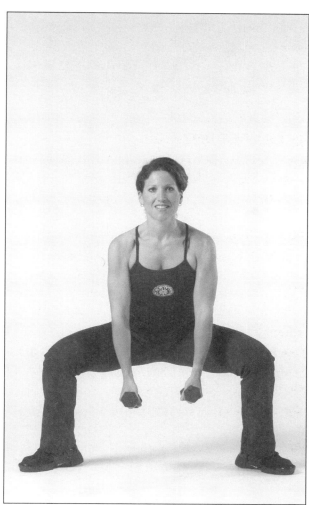

DUMBBELL STIFF-LEGGED DEADLIFTS

This exercise targets both the hamstring muscles at the back of your legs and your lower back muscles. However, if you suffer from lower back injury, this exercise is not recommended because it may harm an already-injured back because of the strain it places on the back muscles. For a machine equivalent, try the Lying Leg Curl Machine.

TECHNIQUE AND FORM

1 Stand in neutral position, with a weight in each hand, your feet shoulder width apart pointing straight ahead, and your legs locked out.

2 Bend from your waist, keeping your legs locked out and your arms hanging down in front of your thighs. Your palms should be turned toward your body.

3 Look straight ahead as you bend over. Lower until your upper body is parallel to the floor and the dumbbells are below your knees.

4 Slowly straighten to the starting position.

TRAINER'S TIPS

It is essential that you keep your back flat as a table as you lower. Pulling your abdominals in and looking straight ahead will help you to maintain proper form.

Use the power of your mind to focus on the hamstrings—think about the back of your legs as you work them.

DUMBBELL
STIFF-LEGGED DEADLIFTS

ONE-LEGGED DUMBBELL CALF RAISES

This exercise can be performed on the floor, but for optimal range of motion, perform it off of a step or bench. Try the Calf Raise Machine as a machine alternate to this exercise.

TECHNIQUE AND FORM

1 Grasp a dumbbell in each hand and position the balls of your right foot on a calf block or a raised platform with the heels extending off. The toes should be facing forward.

2 Lift the left leg to the rear by bending at the knee. This will be your starting position.

3 Raise the heels of your right leg by extending the ankles as high as possible as you contract the calves. Exhale as you perform this movement and contract at the top for a second.

4 Lower the heels by bending the ankles until the calves are fully stretched. Inhale as you perform this portion of the movement.

5 Repeat for the recommended amount of repetitions. When you are done with the right leg, perform the exercise with the left leg.

TRAINER'S TIPS

If you need help balancing, hold a dumbbell in one hand only and place your free hand on a fixed object such as a beam on a squat rack.

ONE-LEGGED DUMBBELL CALF RAISES

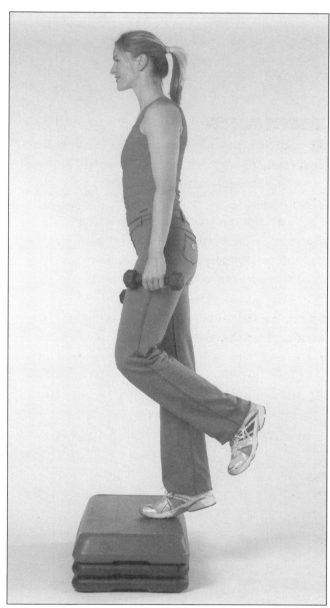

TWO-LEGGED DUMBBELL CALF RAISES

If you perform this exercise on the floor, you won't be able to achieve a full stretch. Using a bench or a step is preferable. For a machine equivalent, try the Calf Raise Machine.

TECHNIQUE AND FORM

1 Stand with your torso upright holding two dumbbells in your hands by your sides. This will be your starting position.

2 With the toes pointing either straight, inwards, or outwards, raise the heels off the floor as you exhale by contracting the calves. Hold the top contraction for a second.

3 As you inhale, go back to the starting position by slowly lowering the heels.

TRAINER'S TIPS

You won't be able to achieve a full stretch at the bottom if you are on the floor. The exercise is effective nonetheless. As you become stronger you may need to use wrist wraps to avoid having the dumbbells slip from your hands.

TWO-LEGGED DUMBBELL CALF RAISES

Chapter 7

Combination Exercises

Get ready for some of the most challenging, heart-pumping exercises you've ever done! While traditional toning exercises focus primarily on one or two muscles groups (for example, the dumbbell row for your mid-back), the combo exercises featured in this chapter work several muscles simultaneously. In most, you will be toning your legs at the same time as you strengthen your upper body. The result? An exercise that efficiently tones your upper and lower body at the same time. And there are additional benefits: because these exercises are all free-weight based, you will be improving balance and strengthening your all-important core muscles as well. As you'll see, the combo exercises are especially suited for an overall body workout that is short on time, but long on intensity.

Because these exercises involve a lot more movement and work more muscles than traditional weight-lifting with machines, you will probably have to use dumbbells that are a bit lighter than you normally would—especially when you first start out. If you find that you are having trouble balancing or performing the exercises in good form, go lighter.

THE **BODY SCULPTING BIBLE** *EXPRESS*

7

SQUATS WITH DUMBBELL ROWS

This exercise pairs the squat for your hamstrings, quadriceps, and gluteals with the row for your back.

TECHNIQUE AND FORM

1 Begin in a standing position, with your body in neutral form, your feet approximately shoulder width apart. Hold a dumbbell in each hand, your arms are down by your sides.

2 Inhale and lower into the squat position with your knees bent, your hips pressed out behind you, and your thighs no lower than parallel to the floor. As you lower yourself, your arms slowly extend in front of your legs at an angle.

3 Exhale and pull your abdominals in toward your spine as you straighten your legs. At the same time as you straighten, bend your arms to bring the weights in toward your waist, pulling your elbows behind you.

4 Extend your arms and lower your body back down into the starting position.

TRAINER'S TIPS

As you begin to lift, make sure that your body weight is balanced over the heels of your feet rather than the toes. A good way to check this is to lift your toes while you are in the squat-ready position to see if you remain balanced. If you can't balance, try shifting your weight back toward your heels.

Your knees should be in line with your toes. It doesn't matter whether your legs are slightly turned out or straight ahead.

Keep your head in line with your spine and look straight ahead as you lift and perform the row.

SQUATS WITH DUMBBELL ROWS

LUNGES WITH OVERHEAD PRESS

You'll feel your heart rate climb with the lunge/overhead press combo, so go easy on the weights—especially if this type of exercise is new to you.

TECHNIQUE AND FORM

1 Stand straight, with a natural curve to your back and a dumbbell in each hand at shoulder height.

2 Step forward with your right leg, bending your right knee until it is perpendicular to the floor. At the same time, bend your left knee behind you, so that it comes close to the floor.

3 As you step forward with your right leg, press the weights up and over your head.

4 Straighten to the starting position, bringing your right leg back to meet your left leg, as you also lower the weights to your shoulders.

5 Repeat beginning with the left leg.

6 Alternate right/left lunges.

TRAINER'S TIPS

◆ Keep your abdominals pulled in tight for this exercise—it will help you remain balanced.

◆ If you feel any sharp pain in your shoulders, switch to lighter weights.

◆ Keep your head straight.

LUNGES WITH OVERHEAD PRESS

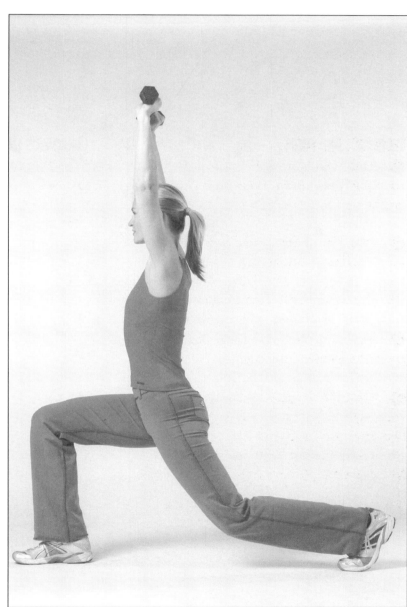

PLIÉ SQUATS WITH TRICEPS EXTENSION

The plié squats with triceps extension works your glutes, your inner and outer thighs, and the backs of your arms.

TECHNIQUE AND FORM

1 Take a wide stance with your legs more than a few feet apart. Bend your legs, pressing your knees to the side.

2 With both hands, hold one weight behind your head, arms bent at your elbows.

3 Exhale and pull your abdominals in toward your spine as you straighten your legs and extend your arms up over your head, pressing the weight toward the ceiling.

4 Hold the top position for a couple of seconds.

5 Lower to start position.

TRAINER'S TIPS

When extending your arms, keep your elbows in by your heard and facing front.

Keep a slight bend in your knees and in your arms, even as you straighten. You don't want to lock out your joints.

PLIÉ SQUATS WITH TRICEPS EXTENSION

KNEE-UP INTO BACK LUNGE WITH BICEPS CURL

This one's like a caffeine rush! Your heart will pump, your legs will feel strong, and your arms will get a great workout. This is a very advanced exercise, so work up to it by performing the lunge/biceps curl without weights until you have good balance.

TECHNIQUE AND FORM

1 Stand straight, with your knees slightly bent and a natural curve to your spine. Hold a weight in each hand by your sides.

2 Exhale as you bring your right knee up in front of you and start to perform alternating biceps curls, beginning with your left arm.

3 Bring your right knee back down and behind your body, so that you are performing a back lunge with your right leg. Bring the knee close to the floor when you lunge.

4 Perform the desired number of reps with the right leg, then switch to the left leg and perform the desired number of reps.

TRAINER'S TIPS

⊗ To modify this exercise if you are a beginner you can perform it without weights or alternate from right to left leg instead of performing consecutive reps with the same leg leading.

⊗ Balance is so important in this exercise. Use your core to pull your abs in tight as you lift your knee up. Ground yourself with your standing leg—concentrate on pressing through the heel of your standing leg to give you support.

KNEE-UP INTO BACK LUNGE WITH BICEPS CURL

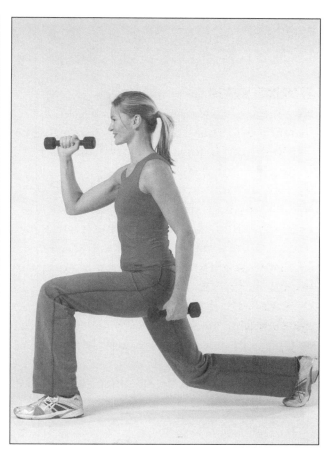

UPRIGHT ROW WITH SIDE-TO-SIDE PLIÉ SQUATS

A great toner for your upper back and legs, this fast moving exercise has cardio benefits too!

TECHNIQUE AND FORM

1 Stand with your knees slightly bent, a weight in each hand at the front of your thighs, and with your palms turned in toward your body.

2 Take a large step to your right and bend your legs so that you are performing a wide plié squat. At the same time as you take the step, bring the weights up to your chest in an upward rowing motion (elbows out to the side).

3 Straighten your legs and pull your left leg in to your body as you lower your weights.

4 Repeat the exercise, this time stepping out to the left as you perform the upright row.

TRAINER'S TIPS

Keep your elbows slightly above the weights as you perform the row.

Lift the weights only as high as your chest or you could injure your shoulders.

UPRIGHT ROW WITH SIDE-TO-SIDE PLIÉ SQUATS

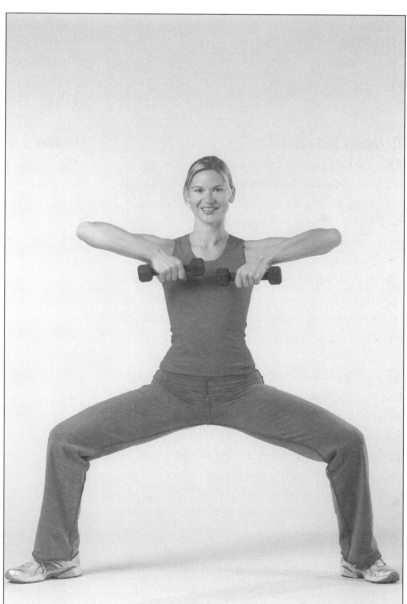

SQUAT WITH ALTERNATING LEG KICK

Control is essential in this great exercise for the heart and legs muscles. Never kick wildly.

TECHNIQUE AND FORM

1 Stand straight, with your knees slightly bent and a slight curve to your spine and your feet approximately shoulder width apart. Hold a dumbbell in each hand and keep your arms down by your sides.

2 Inhale and lower into the squat position with your knees bent, your hips pressed out behind you, and your thighs going no lower than parallel to the floor.

3 Exhale as you straighten your legs. Once they are almost straight, press your left leg out to the side.

4 As you bring your left leg down, immediately perform a squat.

5 Repeat, pressing your right leg out to the side as you come out of the squat.

TRAINER'S TIPS

✪ Think about pressing your leg rather than kicking it—this will help you to use less momentum and more muscle.

✪ You don't have to lift your leg up high to get benefits from this exercise, lift high enough so that you feel a tightening in your outer thighs, but never any sharp pain.

✪ To increase intensity of this exercise you can perform side arm raises with dumbbells as you come out of the squat.

SQUAT WITH ALTERNATING LEG KICK

VARIATION

PUSH-UP WITH SIDE ROTATION

A toughie, this exercise requires significant core (ab/back) strength. Work up to it.

TECHNIQUE AND FORM

1 Face the floor in a push-up-ready position with your arms extended and wider than your chest, your back flat.

2 Bend your arms and lower your chest so that it hovers a couple of inches above the floor.

3 Push back up as you exhale.

4 When you reach the top, lift your right arm off the floor and rotate your body so that you are balancing on your left arm and left foot.

5 Rotate back and return your right hand to the floor, then lower your chest again.

6 Push back up as you exhale, this time lifting your left arm off the floor and rotating your body so that you are balancing on your right side.

TRAINER'S TIPS

To work up to this exercise, begin by performing regular push-ups on bent knees. Progress to performing push-ups with straight legs before adding the rotation.

Think about using your abs and lower back muscles to stabilize your body as you lift. Also think about grounding your body with the opposite arm and leg.

PUSH-UP WITH SIDE ROTATION

DEADLIFT/
ROW COMBO

Perform this exercise for your hamstrings, lower back, and mid-back.

TECHNIQUE AND FORM

1 Stand straight with a weight in each hand.

2 Keeping your back nearly straight, bend at your hips so that the weights are just below your knees. Your palms should face your legs.

3 Exhale and straighten. As you do so, bring the weights in toward your navel, pulling your elbows behind your back to perform a row.

TRAINER'S TIPS

⊘ Proper form is vital to avoid injury to the lower back. Never curve your back when you bend forward. Pulling in your abs tightly can help you to maintain proper form.

⊘ Only go as low as you can in good form.

⊘ When you perform the row, concentrate on squeezing the back muscles for a second or two.

DEADLIFT/ ROW COMBO

Chapter 8
Machine Exercises

As we've mentioned, we prefer that you use dumbbells for your 21-Minute *EXPRESS* Workout whenever possible because of the increased amount of neuromuscular stimulation free weight-based workouts provide. That said, there are times when you may need to choose a machine-based workout—for example, if you are away and your hotel gym has no free weights. There are also times when a machine workout is preferable to a dumbbell version—such as when you have an injury or muscular weakness and you need the extra support a machine provides.

This chapter presents all the machine-based exercises for the *EXPRESS* Workout. The most important thing is to make sure you have proper form and the machine is on the correct settings for your height and fitness level. Since positions vary depending upon machine and manufacturer, carefully read the position instructions that are nearly always posted on the machine.

©2004 Blue Star Creative

8

THE BODY SCULPTING BIBLE
EXPRESS

TWO-ARM ROW MACHINE

BACK AND CHEST EXERCISES

This machine targets the mid-back muscles along with the latissimus dorsi. Secondary emphasis is placed on the trapezius, rhomboids, and biceps brachii muscles. For a similar dumbbell exercise, try the One-Arm Row with either grip.

TECHNIQUE AND FORM

1 Sit on the machine. If it has a pad, position your chest against it. Depending on the machine used, you may need to adjust the length of the chest pad and the height of the seat in a manner that allows your arms to be perpendicular to your torso (at a 90 degree angle) when you grasp the handle bars.

2 Select the desired resistance and grasp the handle bars with a neutral grip (palms facing each other and thumb pointing towards the ceiling). Your arms should be extended in front of you and your shoulders should be stretched. This will be your starting position.

3 Using your back muscles and not your arms, pull the machine lever back towards you until your elbows are past your back and shoulders are pulled back. Hold the contracted position for a second. Breathe out as you perform this movement.

4 Return to the starting position as you breathe in.

TRAINER'S TIPS

It is important that you adjust the machine so that your arms are at a 90 degree angle from your torso in order to maximize back muscle stimulation. If the arms are too high, then the biceps will take the brunt of the work.

Keep control of the machine at all times and concentrate on using the back muscles as opposed to the arms.

The movement can also be performed with a palms down grip or a palms up grip as well. This just slightly changes the angle of stimulation.

©2004 Nautilus, Inc., The Nautilus Group

BENCH PRESS MACHINE

This machine targets the pectoralis major (the mid-chest portion). Secondary emphasis is placed on the clavicular portion of the pectoralis major (upper chest), anterior deltoids, and triceps. For a similar dumbbell exercise, try either a Flat or Incline Dumbbell Bench Press.

TECHNIQUE AND FORM

1 Sit on the machine and adjust the seat of the machine so that your upper chest is placed just above the handle bars provided by the lever.

2 Select the desired resistance and grasp the handle bars with an overhand grip (palms facing down, and thumbs pointing towards each other). Your elbows should be placed out to the sides. The torso, shoulders, and upper arms should be elevated, creating a 90-degree angle between the torso and the upper arms. There should be a straight imaginary line between the bottom of the neck and the elbow.

3 Using your chest muscles and not your arms, push the machine lever away from you until your arms are fully extended in front of you. Hold the contracted position for a second. Breathe out as you perform this movement.

4 Return to the starting position as you breathe in.

TRAINER'S TIPS

The only body parts moving should be the arms as they move the lever forward. The back and head should always remain on the seat. Many people bring the head forward as they perform the movement but this can hyperextend the neck muscles.

Keep control of the machine at all times and concentrate on using the chest muscles as opposed to the arms.

©2004 Blue Star Creative

WIDE GRIP PULLDOWNS TO FRONT

BACK AND CHEST EXERCISES

This machine targets the latissimus dorsi. Secondary emphasis is placed on the midback muscles, trapezius, rhomboids, and biceps brachii muscles. For a similar dumbbell exercise, try the One-Arm Row with either hand grip.

TECHNIQUE AND FORM

1 Select the desired resistance and adjust the height of the thigh supports that prevent the body weight from moving up.

2 Grasp the wide bar on the overhead pulley with an overhand grip (palms facing down) about 3 inches away from shoulder width.

3 With both arms extended in front of you, hold the bar at the chosen grip width, and lean back about 30 degrees while creating a curvature on your lower back and sticking your chest out.

4 As you exhale, pull the bar down until it touches your upper chest by drawing the shoulders and the upper arms down and back. Concentrate on squeezing the back muscles once you reach the fully contracted position and keep the elbows close to your body. The upper torso should remain stationary as you bring the bar to you. Only the arms should move.

5 After a second in the contracted position, breathe in and slowly bring the bar back to the starting position.

TRAINER'S TIPS

Make sure your back and head remain stationary to avoid any type of swinging that could be damaging to the lower back.

Ensure that the bar is taken to the upper chest and not the stomach.

©2004 Blue Star Creative

PECK DECK MACHINE

This machine targets the pectoralis major (the mid chest portion). Secondary emphasis is placed on the clavicular portion of the pectoralis major (upper chest) and anterior deltoids.

TECHNIQUE AND FORM

1 Sit on the machine and adjust the seat so that your upper chest is placed just above the handle bars provided by the lever.

2 Select the desired resistance and grasp the handle bars with a neutral grip (palms facing each other).

3 Position your upper arms in front of you, hands close to each other and upper arms parallel to the floor. This will be your starting position.

4 Move the levers back to the stretched position in which the arms are in line with your torso. Breathe in as you perform this movement.

5 Bring the levers back to the starting position as you exhale and contract the chest muscles. Hold for a second.

TRAINER'S TIPS

⊗ Keep a slight bend to your elbows in order to prevent stress at the biceps tendon.

⊗ Keep your back and the head on the back pad to avoid undue stress on the neck.

⊗ Some machines have handles instead of pads. If this is the case, perform the same movement but with your entire arm parallel to the floor.

©2004 Blue Star Creative

REVERSE FLY MACHINE

SHOULDERS AND ARMS EXERCISES

This machine targets the rear deltoid most effectively. This is one of the few machines which I feel is almost as effective as its free weight version (the Bent-Over Lateral Raise) due to the degree of isolation that it provides.

TECHNIQUE AND FORM

1 Adjust the seat so that the handles are at shoulder height and sit on the machine with your torso pressed against the pad.

2 Grasp the handles.

3 Slightly bend your elbows and rotate your shoulders so that the elbows are to the sides. This is your starting position.

4 Using your rear deltoid muscles, pull the levers apart and to the rear until elbows are just behind back. There should be a slight bend at the elbows. Exhale as you perform this movement and hold the contraction for a second.

5 Slowly return to the starting position as you inhale.

TRAINER'S TIPS

Ensure that the elbows do not drop below the shoulders in order to maximize rear deltoid involvement. If you let the elbows drop, then you start using the back muscles more to perform the movement, thus taking away from deltoid stimulation.

©2004 Nautilus, Inc., The Nautilus Group

LATERAL RAISE MACHINE

This machine targets the side deltoids most effectively.

TECHNIQUE AND FORM

1 Adjust the seat to fit your height and sit on the machine with your back pressed against the pad.

2 Sit on the machine with your arms against the padded levers. Some machines have handles at the end of the pad so grab them if available.

3 Position your elbows to each side of body. This will be your starting position.

4 Using only your side deltoids, raise your arms to each side until your upper arms are parallel to the floor. Exhale as you perform this movement and hold the contraction for a second at the top.

5 Slowly lower the levers and return to the starting position as you inhale.

TRAINER'S TIPS

Perform this exercise slowly as performing it too fast on the way up can injure your shoulders.

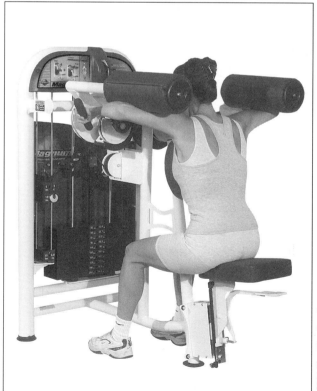

BICEPS CURL MACHINE

This movement targets the biceps brachii with secondary emphasis on the brachialis. For a similar dumbbell exercise, try the Dumbbell Curls.

TECHNIQUE AND FORM

1 Sit on the machine and adjust the seat of the machine so that your upper chest is placed just above the arm pad provided by the machine.

2 Grasp the handles with an underhand grip and position the elbows on top of the arm pad at shoulder width distance. This will be your starting position.

3 Raise the handle bars as you breathe out until the biceps are fully flexed with the back of the upper arm remaining on the pad.

4 Go back to the starting position as you breathe in.

TRAINER'S TIPS

Keep the elbows always in contact with the pad. This will ensure full biceps stimulation.

The upper body should remain stationary as well.

©2004 Nautilus, Inc., The Nautilus Group

TRICEPS EXTENSION MACHINE

This movement targets the triceps brachii. For an equivalent dumbbell exercise, try the Lying Dumbbell Triceps Extension.

TECHNIQUE AND FORM

1 Sit on the machine and adjust the seat of the machine so that your upper chest is placed just above the arm pad provided by the machine.

2 Grasp the handles with a neutral grip (palms facing each other) and position the elbows on top of the arm pad at shoulder width distance. This will be your starting position.

3 Push the lever down until the arm is fully extended. Breathe out as you perform this movement.

4 Go back to the starting position as you breathe in.

TRAINER'S TIPS

Keep the elbows always in contact with the pad. This will ensure full triceps stimulation.

The upper body should remain stationary as well.

HIGH PULLEY CABLE CURLS ON PULLDOWN MACHINE

This movement targets the biceps brachii with secondary emphasis on the brachialis. For a similar dumbbell exercise, try the Dumbbell Curls.

TECHNIQUE AND FORM

1 Stand in front of a pulldown machine with a bar attached to the pulley. If the machine has a bench, simply straddle it.

2 Grab the bar using a shoulder wide grip and position your upper arms in a way that they are parallel to the floor with the palms of the hands facing up. This will be your starting position.

3 Curl the bar towards you until it is close to your forehead. Make sure that as you do so you flex your biceps and exhale. The upper arms should remain stationary and only the forearms should move. Hold for a second on the contracted position.

4 Slowly bring back the arms to the starting position as you inhale.

TRAINER'S TIPS

When you grab the bar before starting the exercise you may slant your torso a bit backwards to maintain good balance.

It is of utmost importance that the upper arms remain stationary as moving them will take off stimulation from the biceps.

©2004 Nautilus Inc., The Nautilus Group

TRICEPS PUSHDOWNS

This movement targets the triceps brachii. For a similar dumbbell exercise, try the Lying Dumbbell Triceps Extension.

TECHNIQUE AND FORM

1 Sit on machine. Grasp handles with your palms facing inward. This is your starting position.

2 Lower the handles until your arms are extended. Your upper arms should remain stationary next to your torso. Only your forearms move. Exhale as you perform this movement.

3 Hold at the contracted position. Then, slowly bring the handles back up to the starting position. Breathe in as you perform this step.

TRAINER'S TIPS

It is of utmost importance that the upper arms remain stationary next to your torso as moving them will take off stimulation from the triceps.

©2004 Blue Star Creative

LYING LEG CURL MACHINE

ABS, LEGS, AND GLUTES EXERCISES

Good isolation machine for the hamstrings. For a similar dumbbell exercise, try the Dumbbell Stiff-Legged Deadlifts.

TECHNIQUE AND FORM

1   Adjust the machine lever to fit your height and lie face down on the leg curl machine (preferably one where the pad is angled as opposed to flat since an angled position is more favorable for hamstrings recruitment) with the pad of the lever on the back of your legs (just a few inches under the calves).

2   Keeping the torso flat on the bench, ensure your legs are fully stretched and grab the side handles of the machine. Position your toes straight. This will be your starting position.

3   As you exhale, curl your legs up as far as possible without lifting the upper legs from the pad. Once you hit the fully contracted position, hold it for a second.

4   As you inhale, bring the legs back to the initial position.

TRAINER'S TIPS

⟡   Never use so much weight that you start using swinging and jerking as you can risk both lower back injury and also a hamstring tear.

LEG EXTENSION MACHINE

ABS, LEGS, AND GLUTES EXERCISES

This is a great machine for isolating the quadriceps muscles. For a similar dumbbell exercise, try the Static Dumbbell Lunges or the Dumbbell Squats.

TECHNIQUE AND FORM

1 Sit on the machine with your legs under the pad and feet pointed forward with your hands holding the side bars. This will be your starting position.

2 Using your quadriceps, extend your legs to the maximum as you exhale. Ensure that the rest of the body remains stationary on the seat. Pause a second on the contracted position.

3 Slowly lower the weight back to the original position as you inhale, ensuring that you do not go past the 90 degree angle limit.

TRAINER'S TIPS

Avoid a fast jerking motion on the way up as that puts undue stress on the kneecaps.

You will need to adjust the pad so that it falls on top of your lower leg (just above your feet). Make sure that your legs form a 90 degree angle between the lower and upper leg. If the angle is less than 90 degrees, then the knee is over the toes which creates undue stress at the knee joint. If the machine is designed that way, make sure that you stop going down once you hit the 90 degree angle.

©2004 Blue Star Creative

LEG PRESS MACHINE

ABS, LEGS, AND GLUTES EXERCISES

Good basic exercise for the legs, albeit not as effective as a squat.

TECHNIQUE AND FORM

1 Using a leg press machine, lie down on the machine and place your legs on the platform directly in front of you at a medium (shoulder width) foot stance. This will be your starting position.

2 As you inhale, slowly lower yourself toward the platform until your upper and lower legs make a 90 degree angle.

3 Pushing mainly with the toes and using the quadriceps, go back to the starting position as you exhale.

TRAINER'S TIPS

If you are using a machine that involves safety bars, exit the machine by getting your legs out first to one side and then your body. Be sure to lock the safety pins properly once you are done. You do not want that platform falling on you fully loaded.

©2004 Blue Star Creative

CALF RAISE MACHINE

ABS, LEGS, AND GLUTES EXERCISES

This movement also targets the gastrocnemius muscle in the calves. For similar dumbbell exercises, try the One- and Two-Legged Calf Raises.

TECHNIQUE AND FORM

1 Adjust the padded lever of the calf raise machine to fit your height.

2 Place your shoulders under the pads provided and position your toes facing forward, inward, or outward. The balls of your feet should be secured on top of the calf block with the heels extending off it. Push the lever up by extending your hips and knees until your torso is standing erect. The knees should be kept with a slight bend and never locked. Toes should be facing forward. This will be your starting position.

3 Raise your heels as you breathe out by extending your ankles as high as possible and flexing your calf. Ensure that the knee is kept stationary at all times. There should be no bending at any time. Hold the contracted position by a second before you start to go back down.

4 Go back slowly to the starting position as you breathe in by lowering your heels as you bend the ankles until calves are stretched.

TRAINER'S TIPS

If you suffer from lower back problems, a better exercise is the calf press. During a standing calf raise the back has to support the weight being lifted.

Maintain your back straight and stationary at all times. Rounding of the back can cause lower back injury.

WIDE-STANCE LEG PRESS (PRESS WITH HEELS) ABS, LEGS, AND GLUTES EXERCISES

This movement targets the gastrocnemius muscle which is the belly of the calves. The machine pictured on the next page is used for both the Wide-Stance Leg Press and the Calf Press exercise.

TECHNIQUE AND FORM

1   Using a leg press machine, sit down on the machine and place your legs high on the platform at a wide stance with toes pointed out at least 45 degrees out.

2   Lower the safety bars holding the weighted platform in place and press the platform all the way up until your legs are fully extended in front of you. (Note: Do not lock your knees.) Your torso and the legs should make perfect 90 degree angle. This will be your starting position.

3   As you inhale, slowly lower the platform until your upper and lower legs bend past a 90 degree angle.

4   Pushing mainly with the heels and using the glutes and hamstrings, go back to the starting position as you exhale.

TRAINER'S TIPS

Do not lock out the knees at the top of the movement as this places undue stress on the knees.

Remember to push with the heel as the purpose is to stimulate the glutes/hamstring tie in on the back of the leg.

Exit the machine by getting your legs out first to one side and then your body. Be sure to lock the safety pins properly once you are done. You do not want that platform falling on you fully loaded.

CALF PRESS

This movement targets the gastrocnemius and soleus muscles of the calves.

TECHNIQUE AND FORM

1 Using a leg press machine, sit down on the machine and place your legs on the platform directly in front of you at a medium (shoulder width) foot stance.

2 Your torso and the legs should make a perfect 90 degree angle. Now carefully place your toes and balls of your feet on the lower portion of the platform with the heels extending off. Toes should be facing forward, outwards, or inwards. This will be your starting position.

3 Press on the platform by raising your heels as you breathe out by extending your ankles as high as possible and flexing your calf. Ensure that the knee is kept stationary at all times. There should be no bending at any time. Hold the contracted position by a second before you start to go back down.

4 Go back slowly to the starting position as you breathe in by lowering your heels as you bend the ankles until calves are stretched.

TRAINER'S TIPS

Make sure you don't use weight that is too heavy or you will strain your knees.

Part III
The Workouts

This part contains the 21-Day Challenge specially designed to jumpstart your exercise program. We also give you two six-week *EXPRESS* Workouts, one featuring dumbbell-only exercises an done using stack machines. You will find optional workouts that focus on your abs and cardio, and on your lower body, if you would like to work those areas even more intensively.

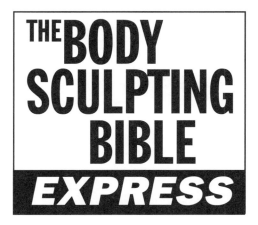

THE **BODY SCULPTING BIBLE**

EXPRESS

Chapter 9
The 21-Day Challenge

THE 21-DAY GET BACK IN SHAPE BODY SCULPTING CHALLENGE!

This routine was written for two types of women: absolute beginners that have never worked out before, and those who have worked out before but have been out of the gym for a while. This routine is guaranteed to firm up your muscles and to burn at the very least 3 to 4 pounds of fat in 21 days, if followed together with the nutrition program recommended in the book. This challenge requires you to perform daily activities that last a maximum of 21 minutes. These activities only require a pair of adjustable dumbbells, a bench or a step, and some sort of cardio-vascular equipment.

After the 21-Day Challenge is completed, then you can graduate to the less time consuming 21-Minute *EXPRESS* Workouts that are presented in the next chapter.

Note: For best results with this program, follow the low calorie plan throughout the duration of the three-week challenge and only have 1 cheat meal on Day 21.

THE BODY SCULPTING BIBLE EXPRESS

9

21-Day Challenge

SPECIAL INSTRUCTIONS: Use Modified Compound Supersets. Perform Modified Compound Supersets by performing the first exercise, resting for the prescribed rest period, performing the second exercise, resting the prescribed rest period, and going back to the first one. Continue in this manner until you have performed all of the prescribed number of sets. Then continue with the next modified compound superset.

MONDAY				DAY 1
EXERCISE	**PAGE NO.**	**REPS**	**SETS**	**REST**
MODIFIED COMPOUND SUPERSET # 1				
Back: One-Arm Rows (Palms facing Torso)	52	18-20	2	60 seconds
Chest: Incline Dumbbell Bench Press	54	18-20	2	60 seconds
MODIFIED COMPOUND SUPERSET # 2				
Thighs: Dumbbell Squats	86	18-20	2	60 seconds
Hamstrings: Dumbbell Stiff-Legged Deadlifts	92	18-20	2	60 seconds

TUESDAY				DAY 2
EXERCISE	**PAGE NO.**	**REPS**	**SETS**	**REST**
Lower Abs: Lying Leg Raises	72	18-20	2	60 seconds
Aerobic Activity				
13 minutes of fast paced walking, stationary bike, or any other type of aerobic activity that you like.				

WEDNESDAY				DAY 3
EXERCISE	**PAGE NO.**	**REPS**	**SETS**	**REST**
MODIFIED COMPOUND SUPERSET # 1				
Shoulders: Dumbbell Upright Rows	62	18-20	2	60 seconds
Calves: Two-Legged Dumbbell Calf Raises	96	18-20	2	60 seconds
MODIFIED COMPOUND SUPERSET # 2				
Biceps: Dumbbell Curls	66	18-20	2	60 seconds
Triceps: Lying Dumbbell Triceps Extensions	68	18-20	2	60 seconds

Week 1

THURSDAY				DAY 4
EXERCISE	PAGE NO.	REPS	SETS	REST
Upper Abs: Crunches	74	18-20	2	60 seconds
Aerobic Activity				
13 minutes of fast paced walking, stationary bike, or any other type of aerobic activity that you like.				

FRIDAY				DAY 5
EXERCISE	PAGE NO.	REPS	SETS	REST
MODIFIED COMPOUND SUPERSET # 1				
Back and Thighs: Squats with Dumbbell Rows	100	18-20	2	60 seconds
Chest and Core: Push-Ups with Side Rotation	112	18-20	2	60 seconds
MODIFIED COMPOUND SUPERSET # 2				
Shoulders and Thighs: Upright Rows with Side-to-Side Plié Squats	108	18-20	2	60 seconds
Triceps and Thighs: Plié Squats with Triceps Extension	104	18-20	2	60 seconds

SATURDAY				DAY 6
EXERCISE	PAGE NO.	REPS	SETS	REST
Lower Abs: Lying Leg Raises	72	18-20	2	60 seconds
Aerobic Activity				
13 minutes of fast paced walking, stationary bike, or any other type of aerobic activity that you like.				

SUNDAY				DAY 7
EXERCISE	PAGE NO.	REPS	SETS	REST
Upper Abs: Crunches	74	18-20	2	60 seconds
Aerobic Activity				
13 minutes of fast paced walking, stationary bike, or any other type of aerobic activity that you like.				

21-Day Challenge

SPECIAL INSTRUCTIONS: Use Modified Compound Supersets. Perform Modified Compound Supersets by performing the first exercise, resting for the prescribed rest period, performing the second exercise, resting the prescribed rest period and going back to the first one. Continue in this manner until you have performed all of the prescribed number of sets. Then continue with the next modified compound superset.

MONDAY				DAY 8
EXERCISE	PAGE NO.	REPS	SETS	REST
MODIFIED COMPOUND SUPERSET # 1				
Back: One-Arm Rows (Palms facing Torso)	52	15-18	3	45 seconds
Chest: Incline Dumbbell Bench Press	54	15-18	3	45 seconds
MODIFIED COMPOUND SUPERSET # 2				
Thighs: Dumbbell Squats	86	15-18	3	45 seconds
Hamstrings: Dumbbell Stiff-Legged Deadlifts	92	15-18	3	45 seconds

TUESDAY				DAY 9
EXERCISE	PAGE NO.	REPS	SETS	REST
Lower Abs: Lying Leg Raises	72	15-18	3	45 seconds
Aerobic Activity				
13 minutes of fast paced walking, stationary bike, or any other type of aerobic activity that you like.				

WEDNESDAY				DAY 10
EXERCISE	PAGE NO.	REPS	SETS	REST
MODIFIED COMPOUND SUPERSET # 1				
Shoulders: Dumbbell Upright Rows	62	15-18	3	45 seconds
Calves: Two-Legged Dumbbell Calf Raises	96	15-18	3	45 seconds
MODIFIED COMPOUND SUPERSET # 2				
Biceps: Dumbbell Curls	66	15-18	3	45 seconds
Triceps: Lying Dumbbell Triceps Extensions	68	15-18	3	45 seconds

Week 2

THURSDAY				DAY 11
EXERCISE	PAGE NO.	REPS	SETS	REST
Upper Abs: Crunches	74	15-18	3	45 seconds
Aerobic Activity				
13 minutes of fast paced walking, stationary bike, or any other type of aerobic activity that you like.				

FRIDAY				DAY 12
EXERCISE	PAGE NO.	REPS	SETS	REST
MODIFIED COMPOUND SUPERSET # 1				
Back and Thighs: Squats with Dumbbell Rows	100	15-18	3	45 seconds
Chest and Core: Push-Ups with Side Rotation	112	15-18	3	45 seconds
MODIFIED COMPOUND SUPERSET # 2				
Shoulders and Thighs: Upright Rows with Side-to-Side Plié Squats	108	15-18	3	45 seconds
Triceps and Thighs: Plié Squats with Triceps Extension	104	15-18	3	45 seconds

SATURDAY				DAY 13
EXERCISE	PAGE NO.	REPS	SETS	REST
Lower Abs: Lying Leg Raises	72	15-18	3	45 seconds
Aerobic Activity				
13 minutes of fast paced walking, stationary bike, or any other type of aerobic activity that you like.				

SUNDAY				DAY 14
EXERCISE	PAGE NO.	REPS	SETS	REST
Upper Abs: Crunches	74	15-18	3	45 seconds
Aerobic Activity				
13 minutes of fast paced walking, stationary bike, or any other type of aerobic activity that you like.				

21-Day Challenge

SPECIAL INSTRUCTIONS: Use Modified Compound Supersets. Perform Modified Compound Supersets by performing the first exercise, resting for the prescribed rest period, performing the second exercise, resting the prescribed rest period and going back to the first one. Continue in this manner until you have performed all of the prescribed number of sets. Then continue with the next modified compound superset.

MONDAY				DAY 15
EXERCISE	**PAGE NO.**	**REPS**	**SETS**	**REST**
MODIFIED COMPOUND SUPERSET # 1				
Back: One-Arm Rows (Palms facing Torso)	52	12-15	4	30 seconds
Chest: Incline Dumbbell Bench Press	54	12-15	4	30 seconds
MODIFIED COMPOUND SUPERSET # 2				
Thighs: Dumbbell Squats	86	12-15	4	30 seconds
Hamstrings: Dumbbell Stiff-Legged Deadlifts	92	12-15	4	30 seconds

TUESDAY				DAY 16
EXERCISE	**PAGE NO.**	**REPS**	**SETS**	**REST**
Lower Abs: Lying Leg Raises	72	12-15	4	30 seconds
Aerobic Activity				
13 minutes of fast paced walking, stationary bike, or any other type of aerobic activity that you like.				

WEDNESDAY				DAY 17
EXERCISE	**PAGE NO.**	**REPS**	**SETS**	**REST**
MODIFIED COMPOUND SUPERSET # 1				
Shoulders: Dumbbell Upright Rows	62	12-15	4	30 seconds
Calves: Two-Legged Dumbbell Calf Raises	96	12-15	4	30 seconds
MODIFIED COMPOUND SUPERSET # 2				
Biceps: Dumbbell Curls	66	12-15	4	30 seconds
Triceps: Lying Dumbbell Triceps Extensions	86	12-15	4	30 seconds

Week 3

THURSDAY				DAY 18
EXERCISE	**PAGE NO.**	**REPS**	**SETS**	**REST**
Upper Abs: Crunches	74	12-15	4	30 seconds
Aerobic Activity				
13 minutes of fast paced walking, stationary bike, or any other type of aerobic activity that you like.				

FRIDAY				DAY 19
EXERCISE	**PAGE NO.**	**REPS**	**SETS**	**REST**
MODIFIED COMPOUND SUPERSET # 1				
Back and Thighs: Squats with Dumbbell Rows	100	12-15	4	30 seconds
Chest and Core: Push-Ups with Side Rotation	112	12-15	4	30 seconds
MODIFIED COMPOUND SUPERSET # 2				
Shoulders and Thighs: Upright Rows with Side-to-Side Plié Squats	108	12-15	4	30 seconds
Triceps and Thighs: Plié Squats with Triceps Extension	104	12-15	4	30 seconds

SATURDAY				DAY 20
EXERCISE	**PAGE NO.**	**REPS**	**SETS**	**REST**
Lower Abs: Lying Leg Raises	72	12-15	4	30 seconds
Aerobic Activity				
13 minutes of fast paced walking, stationary bike, or any other type of aerobic activity that you like.				

SUNDAY				DAY 21
EXERCISE	**PAGE NO.**	**REPS**	**SETS**	**REST**
Upper Abs: Crunches	74	12-15	4	30 seconds
Aerobic Activity				
13 minutes of fast paced walking, stationary bike, or any other type of aerobic activity that you like.				

21-Day Challenge

WEEKLY CHALLENGE			
WEEK	**REPS**	**SETS**	**REST**
WEEK 1	18-20	2	60 SECONDS
WEEK 2	15-18	3	45 SECONDS
WEEK 3	12-15	4	30 SECONDS

MONDAY

MODIFIED COMPOUND SUPERSET # 1

Back: One-Arm Rows (Palms facing Torso)   page 52

Chest: Incline Dumbbell Bench Press   page 54

MODIFIED COMPOUND SUPERSET # 2

Thighs: Dumbbell Squats   page 86

Hamstrings: Dumbbell Stiff-Legged Deadlifts   page 92

TUESDAY/SATURDAY

Lower Abs: Lying   page 72   Cardio
Leg Raises

THURSDAY/SUNDAY

Upper Abs :   page 74   Cardio
Crunches

The Workout

WEDNESDAY

MODIFIED COMPOUND SUPERSET # 1

Shoulders: Dumbbell Upright Rows   page 62

Calves: Two-Legged Dumbbell Calf Raises   page 96

MODIFIED COMPOUND SUPERSET # 2

Biceps: Dumbbell Curls   page 66

Triceps: Lying Dumbbell Triceps Extensions   page 68

MODIFIED COMPOUND SUPERSET # 1

Back and Thighs: Squats with Dumbbell Rows   page 100

Chest and Core: Push-Ups with Side Rotation   page 112

MODIFIED COMPOUND SUPERSET # 2

  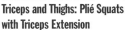

Shoulders and Thighs: Upright   page 108
Rows with Side-to-Side Plié Squats

Triceps and Thighs: Plié Squats   page 104
with Triceps Extension

Chapter 10

The *EXPRESS* Workouts

The Body Sculpting Bible *EXPRESS* program offers three workouts. One is the all-dumbbell workout that can be performed either in the comfort of your home, or at a gym, with an adjustable bench and a set of dumbbells. The second workout is one that makes use of selectorized weight machine equipment (or weight stack machines). This is a good workout to use while on vacation at a hotel gym that does not offer dumbbells. The third is an overall body workout using the combination exercises.

These workouts are designed to be done three days each week within a 21-minute limit. They are fast-paced, providing good cardiovascular conditioning as well as toning and strengthening. On the days off you can perform some abdominal work in the comfort of your home along with some optional cardiovascular exercise.

For the fastest results, you are encouraged to use the dumbbell workout in addition to adding the optional cardiovascular exercise component on your days off.

10

THE **BODY SCULPTING BIBLE** EXPRESS

MONDAY	TUESDAY	WEDNESDAY	THURSDAY	FRIDAY	SATURDAY	SUNDAY
Day 1	Abs/Cardio	Day 2	Abs/Cardio	Day 3	Abs/Cardio	Off
Day 1	Abs/Cardio	Day 2	Abs/Cardio	Day 3	Abs/Cardio	Off

Three days a week weight training with three different routines each week.
Three days of abdominals with optional cardiovascular exercise.

Workout #1: Dumbbell Only

SPECIAL INSTRUCTIONS: Use Modified Compound Supersets. Perform Modified Compound Supersets by doing the exercises and resting the prescribed amount of time until you have completed a circuit. Then start at the beginning and repeat for the recommended number of times before moving on to the next modified compound superset.

ABS AND CARDIO				
EXERCISE	**PAGE NO.**	**REPS**	**SETS**	**REST**
MODIFIED COMPOUND SUPERSET # 1				
Lower Abs: Lying Leg Raises	72	12-15	2	30 seconds
Upper Abs: Crunches	74	12-15	2	30 seconds
Obliques: Bicycle	76	12-15	2	30 seconds
Aerobic Activity				
15 minutes of fast paced walking, stationary bike, or any other type of aerobic activity that you like.				

DAY 1				
EXERCISE	**PAGE NO.**	**REPS**	**SETS**	**REST**
MODIFIED COMPOUND SUPERSET # 1				
Back: One-Arm Rows (Palms facing Torso)	52	12-15	2	30 seconds
Chest: Incline Dumbbell Bench Press	54	12-15	2	30 seconds
Thighs: Dumbbell Squats	86	12-15	2	30 seconds
Hamstrings: Dumbbell Stiff-Legged Deadlifts	92	12-15	2	30 seconds
MODIFIED COMPOUND SUPERSET # 2				
Biceps: Dumbbell Curls	66	12-15	2	30 seconds
Triceps: Lying Dumbbell Triceps Extensions	68	12-15	2	30 seconds
Shoulders: Dumbbell Upright Rows	62	12-15	2	30 seconds
Calves: Two-Legged Dumbbell Calf Raises	96	12-15	2	30 seconds

Weeks 1 & 2

DAY 2				
EXERCISE	**PAGE NO.**	**REPS**	**SETS**	**REST**
MODIFIED COMPOUND SUPERSET # 1				
Thighs: Dumbbell Squats	86	12-15	2	30 seconds
Hamstrings: Static Dumbbell Lunges (Press with Heels)	88	12-15	2	30 seconds
Thighs: Wide-Stance Dumbbell Squats	90	12-15	2	30 seconds
Hamstrings: Dumbbell Stiff-Legged Deadlifts	92	12-15	2	30 seconds
MODIFIED COMPOUND SUPERSET # 2				
Calves: One-Legged Dumbbell Calf Raises	94	12-15	2	30 seconds
Shoulders: Bent-Over Lateral Raises	64	12-15	2	30 seconds
Calves: Two-Legged Dumbbell Calf Raises	96	12-15	2	30 seconds
Triceps: Lying Dumbbell Triceps Extension	68	12-15	2	30 seconds

DAY 3				
EXERCISE	**PAGE NO.**	**REPS**	**SETS**	**REST**
FULL BODY COMBINATION WORKOUT # 1				
Back and Thighs: Squats with Dumbbell Rows	100	12-15	2	30 seconds
Chest and Core: Push-Ups with Side Rotation	112	12-15	2	30 seconds
Shoulders and Thighs: Upright Rows with Side-to-Side Lunges	108	12-15	2	30 seconds
Hamstrings and Back: Deadlift/Row Combo	114	12-15	2	30 seconds
FULL BODY COMBINATION WORKOUT # 2				
Biceps and Thighs: Knee-Ups into Back Lunge with Bicep Curl	106	12-15	2	30 seconds
Triceps and Thighs: Plié Squats with Triceps Extension	104	12-15	2	30 seconds
Shoulders and Thighs: Lunges with Overhead Press	102	12-15	2	30 seconds
Thighs: Squat with Alternating Leg Kick	110	12-15	2	30 seconds

Workout #1: Dumbbell Only

SPECIAL INSTRUCTIONS: Use Supersetting. Perform two exercises with no rest period in between. Rest for 30 seconds and then perform another two exercises with no rest in between. Repeat for the prescribed number of sets and then continue with the next group of exercises.

ABS AND CARDIO

EXERCISE	PAGE NO.	REPS	SETS	REST
MODIFIED COMPOUND SUPERSET # 1				
Lower Abs: Lying Leg Raises	72	10-12	3	0 seconds
Upper Abs: Crunches	74	10-12	3	0 seconds
Obliques: Bicycle	76	10-12	2	30 seconds
Aerobic Activity				
15 minutes of fast paced walking, stationary bike, or any other type of aerobic activity that you like.				

DAY 1

EXERCISE	PAGE NO.	REPS	SETS	REST
MODIFIED COMPOUND SUPERSET # 1				
Back: One-Arm Rows (Palms facing Torso)	52	10-12	3	0 seconds
Chest: Incline Dumbbell Bench Press	54	10-12	3	30 seconds
Thighs: Dumbbell Squats	86	10-12	3	0 seconds
Hamstrings: Dumbbell Stiff-Legged Deadlifts	92	10-12	3	30 seconds
MODIFIED COMPOUND SUPERSET # 2				
Biceps: Dumbbell Curls	66	10-12	3	0 seconds
Triceps: Lying Dumbbell Triceps Extensions	68	10-12	3	30 seconds
Shoulders: Dumbbell Upright Rows	62	10-12	3	0 seconds
Calves: Two-Legged Dumbbell Calf Raises	96	10-12	3	30 seconds

Weeks 3 & 4

DAY 2

EXERCISE	PAGE NO.	REPS	SETS	REST
MODIFIED COMPOUND SUPERSET # 1				
Thighs: Dumbbell Squats	86	10-12	3	0 seconds
Hamstrings: Static Dumbbell Lunges (Press with Heels)	88	10-12	3	30 seconds
Thighs: Wide Stance Dumbbell Squats	90	10-12	3	0 seconds
Hamstrings: Dumbbell Stiff-Legged Deadlifts	92	10-12	3	30 seconds
MODIFIED COMPOUND SUPERSET # 2				
Calves: One-Legged Dumbbell Calf Raises	94	10-12	3	0 seconds
Shoulders: Bent-Over Lateral Raises	64	10-12	3	30 seconds
Calves: Two-Legged Dumbbell Calf Raises	96	10-12	3	0 seconds
Triceps: Lying Dumbbell Triceps Extension	68	10-12	3	30 seconds

DAY 3

EXERCISE	PAGE NO.	REPS	SETS	REST
FULL BODY COMBINATION WORKOUT # 1				
Back and Thighs: Squats with Dumbbell Rows	100	10-12	3	0 seconds
Chest and Core: Push-Ups with Side Rotation	112	10-12	3	30 seconds
Shoulders and Thighs: Upright Rows with Side-to-Side Lunges	108	10-12	3	0 seconds
Hamstrings and Back: Deadlift/Row Combo	114	10-12	3	30 seconds
FULL BODY COMBINATION WORKOUT # 2				
Biceps and Thighs: Knee-Ups into Back Lunge with Bicep Curl	106	10-12	3	0 seconds
Triceps and Thighs: Plié Squats with Triceps Extension	104	10-12	3	30 seconds
Shoulders and Thighs: Lunges with Overhead Press	102	10-12	3	0 seconds
Thighs: Squat with Alternating Leg Kick	110	10-12	3	30 seconds

Workout #1: Dumbbell Only

SPECIAL INSTRUCTIONS: Use Giant Sets. Perform four exercises with no rest period in between. Only rest after the four exercises have been per-formed consecutively. Repeat for the prescribed number of sets and then continue with the next group of exercises.

ABS AND CARDIO

EXERCISE	PAGE NO.	REPS	SETS	REST
GIANT SET # 1				
Lower Abs: Lying Leg Raises	72	8-10	3	0 seconds
Upper Abs: Crunches	74	8-10	3	0 seconds
Obliques: Bicycle	76	8-10	2	30 seconds
Aerobic Activity				
15 minutes of fast paced walking, stationary bike, or any other type of aerobic activity that you like.				

DAY 1

EXERCISE	PAGE NO.	REPS	SETS	REST
GIANT SET # 1				
Back: One-Arm Rows (Palms facing Torso)	52	8-10	3	0 seconds
Chest: Incline Dumbbell Bench Press	54	8-10	3	0 seconds
Thighs: Dumbbell Squats	86	8-10	3	0 seconds
Hamstrings: Dumbbell Stiff-Legged Deadlifts	92	8-10	3	30 seconds
GIANT SET # 2				
Biceps: Dumbbell Curls	66	8-10	3	0 seconds
Triceps: Lying Dumbbell Triceps Extensions	68	8-10	3	0 seconds
Shoulders: Dumbbell Upright Rows	62	8-10	3	0 seconds
Calves: Two-Legged Dumbbell Calf Raises	96	8-10	3	30 seconds

Weeks 5 & 6

DAY 2				
EXERCISE	**PAGE NO.**	**REPS**	**SETS**	**REST**
GIANT SET # 1				
Thighs: Dumbbell Squats	86	8-10	3	0 seconds
Hamstrings: Static Dumbbell Lunges (Press with Heels)	88	8-10	3	0 seconds
Thighs: Wide-Stance Dumbbell Squats	90	8-10	3	0 seconds
Hamstrings: Dumbbell Stiff-Legged Deadlifts	92	8-10	3	30 seconds
GIANT SET # 2				
Calves: One-Legged Dumbbell Calf Raises	94	8-10	3	0 seconds
Shoulders: Bent-Over Lateral Raises	64	8-10	3	0 seconds
Calves: Two-Legged Dumbbell Calf Raises	96	8-10	3	0 seconds
Triceps: Lying Dumbbell Triceps Extension	68	8-10	3	30 seconds

DAY 3				
EXERCISE	**PAGE NO.**	**REPS**	**SETS**	**REST**
FULL BODY COMBINATION GIANT SET # 1 (HEAVIER WEIGHTS)				
Back and Thighs: Squats with Dumbbell Rows	100	8-10	3	0 seconds
Chest and Core: Push-Ups with Side Rotation	112	8-10	3	0 seconds
Shoulders and Thighs: Upright Rows with Side-to-Side Lunges	108	8-10	3	0 seconds
Hamstrings and Back: Deadlift/Row Combo	114	8-10	3	30 seconds
FULL BODY COMBINATION GIANT SET # 1 (HEAVIER WEIGHTS)				
Biceps and Thighs: Knee-Ups into Back Lunge with Bicep Curl	106	8-10	3	0 seconds
Triceps and Thighs: Plié Squats with Triceps Extension	104	8-10	3	0 seconds
Shoulders and Thighs: Lunges with Overhead Press	102	8-10	3	0 seconds
Thighs: Squat with Alternating Leg Kick	110	8-10	3	30 seconds

Workout #2: Machine Only

SPECIAL INSTRUCTIONS: Use Modified Compound Supersets. Perform Modified Compound Supersets by doing the exercises and, resting the prescribed amount of time until you have completed a circuit. Then start at the beginning and repeat for the recommended number of times before moving on to the next modified compound superset.

ABS AND CARDIO				
EXERCISE	**PAGE NO.**	**REPS**	**SETS**	**REST**
MODIFIED COMPOUND SUPERSET # 1				
Lower Abs: Lying Leg Raises	72	12-15	2	30 seconds
Upper Abs: Crunches	74	12-15	2	30 seconds
Obliques: Bicycle	76	12-15	2	30 seconds
Aerobic Activity				
15 minutes of fast paced walking, stationary bike, or any other type of aerobic activity that you like.				

DAY 1				
EXERCISE	**PAGE NO.**	**REPS**	**SETS**	**REST**
MODIFIED COMPOUND SUPERSET # 1				
Back: Two-Arm Row Machine	118	12-15	2	30 seconds
Chest: Bench Press Machine	119	12-15	2	30 seconds
Thighs: Leg Press Machine	130	12-15	2	30 seconds
Hamstrings: Lying Leg Curl Machine	128	12-15	2	30 seconds
MODIFIED COMPOUND SUPERSET # 2				
Biceps: Biceps Curl Machine	124	12-15	2	30 seconds
Triceps: Triceps Extension Machine	125	12-15	2	30 seconds
Shoulders: Lateral Raise Machine	123	12-15	2	30 seconds
Calves: Calf Raise Machine	131	12-15	2	30 seconds

Weeks 1 & 2

DAY 2				
EXERCISE	**PAGE NO.**	**REPS**	**SETS**	**REST**
MODIFIED COMPOUND SUPERSET # 1				
Thighs: Leg Press Machine	130	12-15	2	30 seconds
Hamstrings: Lying Leg Curl Machine	128	12-15	2	30 seconds
Thighs: Leg Extension Machine	129	12-15	2	30 seconds
Hamstrings: Wide-Stance Leg Press (Press with Heels)	132	12-15	2	30 seconds
MODIFIED COMPOUND SUPERSET # 2				
Calves: Calf Raise Machine	131	12-15	2	30 seconds
Shoulders: Lateral Raise Machine	123	12-15	2	30 seconds
Calves: Calf Press	133	12-15	2	30 seconds
Triceps: Triceps Pushdowns	127	12-15	2	30 seconds

DAY 3				
EXERCISE	**PAGE NO.**	**REPS**	**SETS**	**REST**
FULL BODY MODIFIED COMPOUND SUPERSET # 1				
Back: Wide Grip Pulldowns to Front	120	12-15	2	30 seconds
Chest: Peck Deck Machine	121	12-15	2	30 seconds
Thighs: Leg Extension Machine	129	12-15	2	30 seconds
Hamstrings: Wide-Stance Leg Press (Press with Heels)	132	12-15	2	30 seconds
FULL BODY MODIFIED COMPOUND SUPERSET # 2				
Biceps: High Pulley Cable Curls on Pulldown Machine	126	12-15	2	30 seconds
Triceps: Triceps Pushdowns	127	12-15	2	30 seconds
Shoulders: Reverse Fly Machine	122	12-15	2	30 seconds
Calves: Calf Raise Machine	131	12-15	2	30 seconds

Workout #2: Machine Only

SPECIAL INSTRUCTIONS: Use Supersetting. Perform two exercises with no rest period in between. Rest for 30 seconds and then perform another two exercises with no rest in between. Repeat for the prescribed number of sets and then continue with the next group of exercises.

ABS AND CARDIO				
EXERCISE	**PAGE NO.**	**REPS**	**SETS**	**REST**
MODIFIED COMPOUND SUPERSET # 1				
Lower Abs: Lying Leg Raises	72	10-12	3	0 seconds
Upper Abs: Crunches	74	10-12	3	0 seconds
Obliques: Bicycle	76	10-12	2	30 seconds
Aerobic Activity				
15 minutes of fast paced walking, stationary bike, or any other type of aerobic activity that you like.				

DAY 1				
EXERCISE	**PAGE NO.**	**REPS**	**SETS**	**REST**
MODIFIED COMPOUND SUPERSET # 1				
Back: Two-Arm Row Machine	118	10-12	3	0 seconds
Chest: Bench Press Machine	119	10-12	3	30 seconds
Thighs: Leg Press Machine	130	10-12	3	0 seconds
Hamstrings: Lying Leg Curl Machine	128	10-12	3	30 seconds
MODIFIED COMPOUND SUPERSET # 2				
Biceps: Biceps Curl Machine	124	10-12	3	0 seconds
Triceps: Triceps Extension Machine	125	10-12	3	30 seconds
Shoulders: Lateral Raise Machine	123	10-12	3	0 seconds
Calves: Calf Raise Machine	131	10-12	3	30 seconds

Weeks 3 & 4

DAY 2				
EXERCISE	**PAGE NO.**	**REPS**	**SETS**	**REST**
MODIFIED COMPOUND SUPERSET # 1				
Thighs: Leg Press Machine	130	10-12	3	0 seconds
Hamstrings: Lying Leg Curl Machine	128	10-12	3	30 seconds
Thighs: Leg Extension Machine	129	10-12	3	0 seconds
Hamstrings: Wide-Stance Leg Press (Press with Heels)	132	10-12	3	30 seconds
MODIFIED COMPOUND SUPERSET # 2				
Calves: Calf Raise Machine	131	10-12	3	0 seconds
Shoulders: Lateral Raise Machine	123	10-12	3	30 seconds
Calves: Calf Press	133	10-12	3	0 seconds
Triceps: Triceps Pushdowns	127	10-12	3	30 seconds

DAY 3				
EXERCISE	**PAGE NO.**	**REPS**	**SETS**	**REST**
GIANT SET # 1				
Back: Wide Grip Pulldowns to Front	120	10-12	3	0 seconds
Chest: Peck Deck Machine	121	10-12	3	30 seconds
Thighs: Leg Extension Machine	129	10-12	3	0 seconds
Hamstrings: Wide-Stance Leg Press (Press with Heels)	132	10-12	3	30 seconds
GIANT SET # 2				
Biceps: High Pulley Cable Curls on Pulldown Machine	126	10-12	3	0 seconds
Triceps: Triceps Pushdowns	127	10-12	3	30 seconds
Shoulders: Reverse Fly Machine	122	10-12	3	0 seconds
Calves: Calf Raise Machine	131	10-12	3	30 seconds

Workout #2: Machine Only

SPECIAL INSTRUCTIONS: Use Giant Sets. Perform four exercises with no rest period in between. Only rest after the four exercises have been performed consecutively. Repeat for the prescribed number of sets and then continue with the next group of exercises.

ABS AND CARDIO				
EXERCISE	PAGE NO.	REPS	SETS	REST
GIANT SET # 1				
Lower Abs: Lying Leg Raises	72	10-12	3	0 seconds
Upper Abs: Crunches	74	10-12	3	0 seconds
Obliques: Bicycle	76	12-15	2	30 seconds
Aerobic Activity				
15 minutes of fast paced walking, stationary bike, or any other type of aerobic activity that you like.				

DAY 1				
EXERCISE	PAGE NO.	REPS	SETS	REST
GIANT SET # 1				
Back: Two-Arm Row Machine	118	10-12	3	0 seconds
Chest: Bench Press Machine	119	10-12	3	0 seconds
Thighs: Leg Press Machine	130	10-12	3	0 seconds
Hamstrings: Lying Leg Curl Machine	128	10-12	3	30 seconds
GIANT SET # 1				
Biceps: Biceps Curl Machine	124	10-12	3	0 seconds
Triceps: Triceps Extensions Machine	125	10-12	3	0 seconds
Shoulders: Lateral Raise Machine	123	10-12	3	0 seconds
Calves: Calf Press	133	10-12	3	30 seconds

Weeks 5 & 6

DAY 2

EXERCISE	PAGE NO.	REPS	SETS	REST
GIANT SET # 1				
Thighs: Leg Press Machine	130	10-12	3	0 seconds
Hamstrings: Lying Leg Curl Machine	128	10-12	3	0 seconds
Thighs: Leg Extension Machine	129	10-12	3	0 seconds
Hamstrings: Wide-Stance Leg Press (Press with Heels)	132	10-12	3	30 seconds
GIANT SET # 2				
Calves: Calf Raise Machine	131	10-12	3	0 seconds
Shoulders: Lateral Raise Machine	123	10-12	3	0 seconds
Calves: Calf Press	133	10-12	3	0 seconds
Triceps: Triceps Pushdowns	127	10-12	3	30 seconds

DAY 3

EXERCISE	PAGE NO.	REPS	SETS	REST
GIANT SET # 1				
Back: Wide Grip Pulldowns to Front	120	10-12	3	0 seconds
Chest: Peck Deck Machine	121	10-12	3	0 seconds
Thighs: Leg Extension Machine	129	10-12	3	0 seconds
Hamstrings: Wide-Stance Leg Press (Press with Heels)	132	10-12	3	30 seconds
GIANT SET # 2				
Biceps: High Pulley Cable Curls on Pulldown Machine	126	10-12	3	0 seconds
Triceps: Triceps Pushdowns	127	10-12	3	0 seconds
Shoulders: Reverse Fly Machine	122	10-12	3	0 seconds
Calves: Calf Raise Machine	131	10-12	3	30 seconds

Supplemental Workout

SPECIAL INSTRUCTIONS: The *EXPRESS* workout was designed to provide you with an easy to follow, challenging strength training regimen in 21 minutes. In addition, optional cardio/abs workouts are available for your off days. For those of you who may want to focus exclusively on cardio and abdominal work, you can do the following program. Once again you will work four days each week for just 21 minutes a day. You can do this program on its own or in addition to the *EXPRESS* Workout. You also can use the off days of this program to do some of the strength training routines.

WEEKS 1 AND 2

DAY 1

CARDIO: Seventeen minutes of cardiovascular exercise at an intensity that raises your heart rate into the training zone. To determine the training zone simply subtract your age from 220 and work within a range that causes your heart to beat at 60 to 80 percent of the resulting number.

ABDOMINALS/CORE

EXERCISE	PAGE NO.	REPS	SETS	REST
MODIFIED COMPOUND SUPERSET Upper Abs: Crunches	74	12-15	3	15 seconds
Obliques: Bicycle	76	12-15	3	15 seconds
Lower Back: Extension	82	12-15	3	15 seconds

DAY 2

CARDIO: Seventeen minutes of cardiovascular exercise at an intensity that raises your heart rate into the training zone.

ABDOMINALS/CORE

EXERCISE	PAGE NO.	REPS	SETS	REST
MODIFIED COMPOUND SUPERSET Lower Abs: Lying Leg Raises	72	10-12	3	15 seconds
Upper Abs: Crunches	74	10-12	3	15 seconds
Obliques: Bicycle	76	10-12	3	15 seconds
Lower Back: Extension	82	10-12	3	15 seconds

Cardio/Abs Intensive

MONDAY	TUESDAY	WEDNESDAY	THURSDAY	FRIDAY	SATURDAY	SUNDAY
Day 1	Off	Day 2	Off	Day 1	Off	Day 2
Day 1	Off	Day 2	Off	Day 1	Off	Day 2

WEEKS 3 AND 4

DAY 1

CARDIO: Seventeen minutes of cardiovascular exercise at an intensity that raises your heart rate into the training zone. Try to increase the intensity over the previous two weeks by either going faster or working out against resistance (adding hills, climbs, or fast intervals).

ABDOMINALS/CORE

EXERCISE	PAGE NO.	REPS	SETS	REST
MODIFIED COMPOUND SUPERSET				
Lower Abs: Lying Leg Raises	72	8-10	3	0 seconds
Upper Abs: Crunches	74	8-10	3	15 seconds
Obliques: Bicycle	76	8-10	3	0 seconds
Lower Back: Extension	82	8-10	3	15 seconds

DAY 2

CARDIO: Seventeen minutes of cardiovascular exercise at an intensity that raises your heart rate into the training zone. Try to increase the intensity over the previous two weeks by either going faster or working out against resistance (adding hills, climbs, or fast intervals).

ABDOMINALS/CORE

EXERCISE	PAGE NO.	REPS	SETS	REST
MODIFIED COMPOUND SUPERSET				
Lower Abs: Lying Leg Raises	72	8-10	3	0 seconds
Upper Abs: Crunches	74	8-10	3	15 seconds
Obliques: Bicycle	76	8-10	3	0 seconds
Overall Core: Plank	78	3 *(hold centered for 10 seconds, left arm/right leg extended for 5 seconds, then right arm/left leg extended for 5 seconds)*	3	15 seconds

Supplemental Workout:
Cardio/Abs Intensive
WEEKS 5 AND 6

DAY 1

CARDIO: Seventeen minutes of cardiovascular exercise at an intensity that raises your heart rate into the training zone. Try speed intervals, in which you go at a very intense level for one minute and then reduce your speed for the next minute, then increase it again for a minute; continue alternating until you've completed the 17 minutes.

ABDOMINALS/CORE

EXERCISE	PAGE NO.	REPS	SETS	REST
MODIFIED COMPOUND SUPERSET Lower Abs: Lying Leg Raises	72	8-10	3	0 seconds
Upper Abs: Crunches	74	8-10	3	0 seconds
Obliques: Bicycle	76	8-10	3	0 seconds
Lower Back: Extension	82	8-10	3	15 seconds

DAY 2

CARDIO: Seventeen minutes of cardiovascular exercise at an intensity that raises your heart rate into the training zone. Try speed intervals, in which you go at a very intense level for one minute and then reduce your speed for the next minute, then increase it again for a minute; continue alternating until you've completed the 17 minutes.

ABDOMINALS/CORE

EXERCISE	PAGE NO.	REPS	SETS	REST
MODIFIED COMPOUND SUPERSET Lower Abs: V-Knee	80	8-10	3	0 seconds
Upper Abs: Crunches	74	8-10	3	0 seconds
Obliques: Bicycle	76	8-10	3	0 seconds
Overall Core: Plank	78	3 *(hold centered for 10 seconds, left arm/right leg extended for 5 seconds, then right arm/left leg extended for 5 seconds)*	3	15 seconds

Supplemental Workout:
Lower Body

SPECIAL INSTRUCTIONS: For those of you who really want to concentrate on toning your legs, here's a supplemental workout you can perform. This workout can be done in addition to the others in any of the other programs we presented, or in place of an upper body workout. The supersets in this workout involve performing several exercises for a single muscle group without resting, and then repeating the sequence for the desired number of sets. To increase the intensity of the workout, increase the weight you're lifting every two weeks.

SUPPLEMENTAL LOWER BODY WORKOUT

EXERCISE	PAGE NO.	REPS	SETS	REST
MODIFIED COMPOUND SUPERSET # 1				
Quads and Glutes: Dumbbell Squats	86	12-15	3	0 seconds
Quads and Glutes: Wide-Stance Dumbbell Squats	90	12-15	3	0 seconds
Quads and Glutes: Leg Press Machine	130	12-15	3	30 seconds
MODIFIED COMPOUND SUPERSET # 2				
Quads and Glutes: Static Dumbbell Lunges	88	12-15	3	0 seconds
Hamstrings: Dumbbell Stiff-Legged Deadlifts	92	12-15	3	0 seconds
Calves: Calf Raise Machine	131	12-15	3	30 seconds
MODIFIED COMPOUND SUPERSET # 3				
Quads: Leg Extension Machine	129	12-15	3	0 seconds
Hamstrings: Lying Leg Curl Machine	128	12-15	3	30 seconds

Appendix A
Training Journal

A

Research has shown that keeping a journal of your daily activity is a great way to ensure that you are meeting your exercise goals. Use the Body Sculpting Bible *EXPRESS* Training Journal to keep track of your progress.

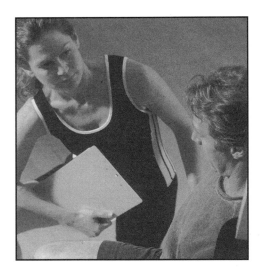

THE BODY SCULPTING BIBLE EXPRESS

BREAK-IN ROUTINE #1

Daily Workout Journal   Week ◯   Day ◯

	Exercise Main (Alternate)	Rest	Set 1 Reps	Set 1 Weight	Set 2 Reps	Set 2 Weight	Set 3 Reps	Set 3 Weight
Superset or Giant Set 1								
Superset or Giant Set 2								
Superset or Giant Set 1								
Superset or Giant Set 2								
Abs								

Cardio

Cardio Activity: _____   Notes: _____

Average Heart Rate: _____

Duration: _____

Appendix B

Food Charts and Nutrition

Good nutrition boils down to some simple basics:

Always try to use natural foods. Avoid using canned or prepared foods as they usually contain too much fat, sodium, and carbs.

Stay within plus or minus 10 grams of the recommended amount of carbs and proteins, plus or minus five grams for fats.

Always choose low-fat protein sources. Don't worry about incurring a fat deficiency since the supplements program takes care of the need for essential fatty acids. Besides, there are trace amounts of fats even in low-fat protein sources.

If you choose to include skim milk in your diet, remember that it not only has protein but also simple carbs. Therefore, count milk as both. Since the carbs in milk are simple carbs, this should only be used in the post workout meal. However, if you schedule requires you to include more protein shakes throughout the day, and you will rely on the carbs in skim milk, add a teaspoon of flaxseed oil to the milk to slow down the release of simple carbs into the bloodstream.

Try to include fibrous carbs in at least two meals.

THE BODY SCULPTING BIBLE EXPRESS

B

Daily Nutrition Journal   Week ◯ Day ◯

	Food	Serving Size	Calories	Carbs (grams)	Protein (grams)	Fat (grams)
Meal 1						
Meal 2						
Meal 3						
Meal 4						
Meal 5						
Meal 6						
TOTAL						

Use the Daily Nutrition Journal to keep track of your diet. Photocopy the page as many times as you need.

1200-CALORIE WEEKS

MEAL 1 (7:30 a.m.)   BREAKFAST (post-workout)
Choose 24 grams from Group A
Choose 24 grams from Group C

MEAL 2 (10:30 a.m.)   MORNING BREAK SNACK
Choose 24 grams from Group A
Choose 24 grams from Group B

MEAL 3 (1:30 p.m.)   LUNCH TIME
Choose 24 grams from Group A
Choose 19 grams from Group B
Choose 5 grams from Group D

MEAL 4 (3:30 p.m.)   AFTERNOON BREAK SNACK
Choose 24 grams from Group A
Choose 24 grams from Group B

MEAL 5 (6:30 p.m.)   DINNER
Choose 24 grams from Group A
Choose 14 grams from Group B
Choose 10 grams from Group D

NOTE: Include one tsp of olive oil three times a day with any meals (except the post-workout meal) on one day. The next day, include one tsp of olive oil once a day and one tsp of flaxseed oil twice a day with any meals (except the post workout meal). This in conjunction with the naturally occurring fats in the food will cover your essential fats needs.

1500-CALORIE WEEKS

MEAL 1 (7:30 a.m.)   BREAKFAST (post-workout)
Choose 25 grams from Group A
Choose 25 grams from Group C

MEAL 2 (10:30 a.m.)   MORNING BREAK SNACK
Choose 25 grams from Group A
Choose 25 grams from Group B

MEAL 3 (12:30 p.m.)   LUNCH TIME
Choose 25 grams from Group A
Choose 20 grams from Group B
Choose 5 grams from Group D

MEAL 4 (3:30 p.m.)   AFTERNOON BREAK SNACK
Choose 25 grams from Group A
Choose 25 grams from Group B

MEAL 5 (6:30 p.m.)   DINNER
Choose 25 grams from Group A
Choose 15 grams from Group B
Choose 10 grams from Group D

MEAL 6 (8:30 p.m.)   LATE SNACK
Choose 25 grams from Group A
Choose 15 grams from Group B
Choose 10 grams from Group D

NOTE: Include one tsp of olive oil three times a day with any meals (except the post workout meal) on one day. The next day, include one tsp of olive oil once a day and one tsp of flaxseed oil twice a day with any meals (except the post workout meal). This in conjunction with the naturally occurring fats in the food will cover your essential fats needs.

FOOD GROUP TABLES

For the post-workout meal, choose one item from Group A and one item from Group C in order to create a balanced meal. For all other meals, choose one item from Group A, one item from Group B, and one item from Group D. Remember to adjust the serving size depending upon the amount of nutrients that you require per meal.

GROUP A - PROTEIN			
FOOD	GRAMS	FOOD	GRAMS
Chicken breast (3.5 oz broiled)	33	White fish (3.5 oz broiled)	31
Tuna (packed in water, 3.5 oz)	35	Halibut (3.5 oz broiled)	31
Turkey breast (3.5 oz broiled)	28	Cod (3.5 oz broiled)	31
Whey protein powder (2 scoops)	22	Round steak (3.5 oz broiled)	33
10 egg whites	35	Top sirloin (4 oz)	35

Note: These weights are for uncooked portions

GROUP B - CARBOHYDRATE (COMPLEX, STARCHY)			
FOOD	GRAMS	FOOD	GRAMS
Baked potato (3.5 oz broiled)	21	Lentils (1 cup dry, cooked)	38
Plain oatmeal (1/2 cup dry)	27	Grits (1/4 cup dry)	31
Whole wheat bread (1 slice; limit if reducing body fat)	13	Pita bread (1 piece)	33
Cream of rice (1/4 cup dry, post workout only)	38	Sweet potato (4 oz)	28
Chickpeas (1 cup cooked)	45	Brown rice (2/3 cup cooked)	30

GROUP C - CARBOHYDRATE (SIMPLE)			
FOOD	GRAMS	FOOD	GRAMS
Apple (1)	15	Banana (6 oz, *post workout only*)	27
Cantaloupe (1/2)	25	Grapes (1 cup, *post workout only*)	14
Strawberries (1 cup)	9	Grapefruit (1/2)	12
Orange (1)	15	Tangerine (1)	9
Pear (1)	27	Cherries (1 cup)	22
Lemon (1)	5	Nectarine (1)	16
Peach (1)	10	Skim milk (1 cup, *preferably post workout only*)	13

GROUP D - CARBOHYDRATE (COMPLEX, FIBROUS)			
FOOD (10 OZ SERVING)	GRAMS	FOOD (10 OZ SERVING)	GRAMS
Asparagus	5	Yellow squash	12
Broccoli	17	Green beans	23
Cabbage	6	Cauliflower	12
Celery	6	Cucumber	7
Mushrooms	6	Lettuce	7
Red or Green peppers	15	Tomato	5
Spinach	3	Zucchini	13

Appendix C
Useful Resources

WWW.BODYSCULPTINGBIBLE.COM

A powerful resource for anyone seeking advice knowledge and more. Loaded with news, fitness tips, and discussion forums, this is a must see.

WWW.HRFIT.NET

A visit here will reward you with a well-rounded bushel of information written by Hugo Rivera, ranging from how to design a workout routine to how to select or reject a food supplement.

WWW.BODYBUILDING.COM

Tons of free information on anything you need to know about bodybuilding and fitness written by several experts in the industry. They also carry most supplement brands in the market selling them at a huge discount.

WWW.POWERBLOCKS.COM

Home of the PowerBlocks™, here you will find the world's most efficient dumbbells in terms of space and feasibility of changing the weights.

WWW.FITNESSFACTORY.COM

A great place to fulfill your home gym equipment needs. They have awesome customer service and great prices.

WWW.PROLAB.COM

Homepage of our recommended line of supplements. They carry all of the basic supplements that bodybuilders need. In addition, all of their supplements are produced with state-of-the-art manufacturing and are sold at the right price.

WWW.INFINITYFITNESS.COM

Website of training and nutrition consultant Scott Mendelson. Scott is a super knowledgeable guy who has tons of free information on his site. He also carries state-of-the-art products.

WWW.DAVEDRAPER.COM

Dave is a bodybuilding legend. Winner of the Mr. America, Mr. World, and Mr. Universe, Dave shares his extensive knowledge in a very straightforward, simple, and almost poetic manner.

WWW.MUSCLEBUILDINGDIET.COM

Owned by Todd Mendelsohn, a former Mr. Central Florida who works as a nutrition/training consultant. If you want more advanced tailor made programs for bulking up, this is the place to go.

Bonus Recipes
for a **Stronger** *more*
Sculpted Body!

A Note from Chef Marie

Following are 60 Breakfast, Lunch, Dinner and Dessert recipes. All of these recipes meet the requirements for nutritious, low-fat weight loss and, when used in conjunction with the 21-Day *EXPRESS* Body Sculpting program, are guaranteed to produce results.

How to Begin

At the start of each week, use the Daily Nutrition Journal in Appendix B to outline your meal plans. You can pick and choose your weekly meals from each category; just be sure that your daily caloric requirement is within the right range for weight loss (1200-1500).

Also, as explained on page 25, keep in mind that, during the first two weeks of your workout, you should aim to consume 1200 calories, and then increase your caloric intake to 1500 calories for the last 2 weeks. This will help your body gain muscle and lose fat more efficiently.

If you prefer to prepare your meals entirely on your own, consult the nutrition guidelines and use the food group charts in Appendix B as a guide.

A Note on Sunday Rewards

If you've stayed true to your diet all week, you deserve a reward. Treat yourself to one "cheat meal" per week. As described on pages 31-32, this can include an appetizer, main meal, and dessert. But be sure not to go overboard, or you'll run the risk of going backwards.

A Note on Times to Eat and Frequency of Meals

To help boost your metabolism, you should try to eat five or six small meals throughout the day, which amounts to approximately every 2-3 hours. This will make it easier for your body to get the energy it needs to build muscle and burn fat.

Choosing Healthier Food for Better Health

You should always try to use fresh and organic products. Limiting the amount of chemicals, colorings, preservatives, and additives in your food will benefit your body and decrease the chances of food allergies, sensitivities, and diseases.

Use canola oil, olive oil, and grapeseed oil (a great substitution to butter because of its buttery flavor) which are the healthiest fats for cooking. Those oils, plus flaxseed oil, fish oil, and walnut oil should be used for salads or cold applications. Remember that these are still fats, and you should use as little as possible which is already done in these recipes.

Reduce animal proteins and increase plant proteins such as beans or tofu. Quickly par-boil or steam vegetables to preserve their vitamins and minerals, which will also limit the addition of calories that are often found in casseroles or other vegetable dishes.

Use low-sodium and low-fat broth/stock for light sauces rather than using fats such as butter, cream, or beurre manié (butter and flour combination). Thicken sauces with cornstarch/arrowroot or waxy maze (for frozen dishes as it won't separate) instead of using flour or a flour-butter mixture. As many of these recipes are low in fat, which we know contributes to flavor, try adding flavor with fresh herbs, spices, and vegetable-concentrated broth/stock. Remember that a pinch of salt can go a long way. Way too many recipes use too much salt, which is harmful to your health because it increases blood pressure, and isn't necessary to obtain a well-balanced recipe. ■

Chef Marie-Annick Courtier is a native of Paris, France, where she learned about gourmet foods and wine in the French tradition. Chef Marie holds a Culinary Arts Degree, has worked with many world renowned chefs, and runs her own personal chef service. A Certified Fitness Nutritionist and Professional Food Manager, she also teaches cooking and created the new Certified Personal Fitness Chef Program. Chef Marie lives in Orange County, California.

One of the most important (and most commonly overlooked) aspects of a healthy diet is proper hydration. As explained on page 30, you can use the formula (0.66 x body weight) to figure out how many ounces of water you need to drink throughout the day.

Breakfast

Y ou have probably heard the phrase "breakfast is the most important meal of the day" many times. With the hectic pace of life today, stopping to eat on your way out the door can seem like a chore. But if you don't take the time to eat first thing in the morning, you will throw off your eating regimen for the rest of the day, and risk undoing all your hard work at the gym!

Be sure to eat breakfast no later than 30 minutes after you wake up. The recipes below are designed to kickstart your day and provide you with the physical and mental energy you will need to get through the morning. Stick to it and you will notice that the first part of your day is a lot easier to handle when you provide your body with the nutrients it needs. Your energy boost is sure to increase your productivity—and encourage your metabolism to work fast, so that the pounds come off easier.

Oatmeal with Mango and Kiwi

Yield: 1 serving

    1/2 cup to 3/4 cup oatmeal
    1   cup to 1½ cup low-fat milk, hot
    1   teaspoon almonds
    1/4 mango, diced
    1   kiwi, diced

Mix the oatmeal with the hot milk until the liquid is incorporated. Add in the almonds, mango, kiwi, and serve immediately.

Option: Add 1 scoop protein powder which adds 100 calories

Per Serving (1/2 cup oatmeal): 356 Cal (18% from Fat, 15% from Protein, 67% from Carb); 14 g Protein; 7 g Tot Fat; 3 g Sat Fat; 2 g Mono Fat; 63 g Carb; 9 g Fiber; 29 g Sugar; 340 mg Calcium; 2 mg Iron; 105 mg Sodium; 20 mg Cholesterol
Per Serving (3/4 cup oatmeal): 483 Cal (18% from Fat, 16% from Protein, 66% from Carb); 21 g Protein; 10 g Tot Fat; 5 g Sat Fat; 3 g Mono Fat; 84 g Carb; 11 g Fiber; 35 g Sugar; 490 mg Calcium; 2 mg Iron; 156 mg Sodium; 29 mg Cholesterol

Homemade Granola with Berries

Yield: 7 to 10 servings

    1/4 cup honey
    1/4 cup vegetable oil
    1   teaspoon vanilla extract
    3 ½ cup old fashioned oats, uncooked
    1/4 cup sliced almonds
    1/4 cup pumpkin seeds
    1/4 cup raisins
    1/4 cup cranberries
    2   teaspoons cinnamon

Preheat the oven to 350°F.
    In a bowl, mix the honey, oil, vanilla extract, and cinnamon. Stir in the oats, almonds, pumpkin seeds, raisins, and cranberries. Mix well and spread over a greased cookie sheet. Bake for 10 minutes. Stir and continue to bake for another 10 minutes or until golden brown. Cool completely and break apart.

Option: Add 1 scoop protein powder which adds 100 calories

Per Serving (1/2 cup homemade granola 1/2 cup low-fat milk, 1/4 cup mixed fresh berries, and 1 teaspoon freshly grinded flaxseeds): 424 Cal (30% from Fat, 14% from Protein, 56% from Carb); 15 g Protein; 15 g Tot Fat; 3 g Sat Fat; 4 g Mono Fat; 61 g Carb; 10 g Fiber; 19 g Sugar; 202 mg Calcium; 3 mg Iron; 54 mg Sodium; 10 mg Cholesterol
Per Serving (3/4 cup homemade granola, 3/4 cup low-fat milk, 1/4 cup mixed fresh berries, and 1 teaspoon freshly grinded flaxseeds): 604 Cal (30% from Fat, 14% from Protein, 56% from Carb); 22 g Protein; 20 g Tot Fat; 5 g Sat Fat; 6 g Mono Fat; 87 g Carb; 13 g Fiber; 28 g Sugar; 295 mg Calcium; 5 mg Iron; 80 mg Sodium; 15 mg Cholesterol

Kashi Flakes with Apples and Walnuts

Yield: 1 serving

1/2 to 3/4 cup Kashi Seven Whole Grains Flakes
1/2 to 3/4 cup low-fat milk, hot or cold
1/4 cup apples
1 tablespoon walnuts
1 teaspoon flaxseeds
Cinnamon to taste

In a bowl mix the cereal with the milk and cinnamon. Top with the apples and walnuts. Sprinkle the freshly ground flaxseeds and serve immediately.

Option: Add 1 scoop protein powder which adds 100 calories

Per Serving (1/2 cup Kashi and 1/2 cup low-fat milk): 228 Cal (33% from Fat, 15% from Protein, 53% from Carb); 9 g Protein; 9 g Tot Fat; 2 g Sat Fat; 2 g Mono Fat; 32 g Carb; 2 g Fiber; 12 g Sugar; 158 mg Calcium; 2 mg Iron; 126 mg Sodium; 10 mg Cholesterol
Per Serving (3/4 cup Kashi and 3/4 cup low-fat milk): 303 Cal (29% from Fat, 15% from Protein, 56% from Carb); 12 g Protein; 10 g Tot Fat; 3 g Sat Fat; 2 g Mono Fat; 45 g Carb; 2 g Fiber; 16 g Sugar; 229 mg Calcium; 3 mg Iron; 189 mg Sodium; 15 mg Cholesterol

Fennel, Leek, and Spinach Omelette

Yield: 1 serving

1/2 teaspoon canola oil
2 to 3 eggs (or 1/2 cup to 3/4 cup egg beaters)
1 tablespoon low-fat milk
3 ounces leek, white part only and thinly sliced
3 ounces fennel bulb, thinly sliced (about 1/2 small bulb)
1/4 cup spinach, thinly sliced
Pinch nutmeg
Salt and pepper to taste

Heat the oil in a nonstick pan over medium heat. Add the leek, fennel, and sauté until tender, about 3 minutes. Add the spinach, lightly season, and sauté another minute or two.

Meanwhile, beat the eggs in a bowl and lightly season to taste. Mix in the nutmeg and pour the mixture into a nonstick pan. Cook until the base of the omelette has set and spread over the cooked vegetables evenly. Reduce heat and continue to cook until almost completely set, about 2 to 3 minutes. Fold over in half, cook for another minute, and serve immediately.

Per Serving (2 eggs): 280 Cal (47% from Fat, 25% from Protein, 29% from Carb); 18 g Protein; 15 g Tot Fat; 4 g Sat Fat; 6 g Mono Fat; 20 g Carb; 4 g Fiber; 5 g Sugar; 179 mg Calcium; 5 mg Iron; 236 mg Sodium; 492 mg Cholesterol
Per Serving (3 eggs): 365 Cal (50% from Fat, 27% from Protein, 23% from Carb); 25 g Protein; 20 g Tot Fat; 6 g Sat Fat; 8 g Mono Fat; 21 g Carb; 4 g Fiber; 6 g Sugar; 210 mg Calcium; 6 mg Iron; 317 mg Sodium; 737 mg Cholesterol

Scrambled Eggs with Tomatoes & Onions

Yield: 1 serving

1   teaspoon olive oil
3   ounces yellow onion, chopped (about 1/2 medium onion)
4   ounces plum tomatoes; peeled, seeded, and chopped (about 1 large tomato)
3   ounces eggplant, skin removed and diced (about 1/2 medium eggplant)
1   garlic clove, minced
1   tablespoon freshly minced basil
2 to 3 eggs (or 1/2 cup to 3/4 cup egg beaters)
Salt and pepper to taste

Heat the oil in a nonstick pan over medium heat. Add the onion and sauté until translucent. Add the tomatoes, eggplant, garlic, and cook until all liquid evaporates.

Beat the eggs in a bowl with the basil and season to taste. Pour the eggs over the vegetables. Cook over medium heat, stirring and scraping the bottom and sides of the pan constantly with a wooden spoon. As soon as the eggs begin to set, remove from heat, continue to stir for a few seconds, and serve immediately.

Per Serving (2 eggs): 292 Cal (50% from Fat, 23% from Protein, 27% from Carb); 17 g Protein; 17 g Tot Fat; 4 g Sat Fat; 8 g Mono Fat; 20 g Carb; 6 g Fiber; 10 g Sugar; 108 mg Calcium; 3 mg Iron; 173 mg Sodium; 491 mg Cholesterol
Per Serving (3 eggs): 377 Cal (53% from Fat, 26% from Protein, 21% from Carb); 25 g Protein; 22 g Tot Fat; 6 g Sat Fat; 10 g Mono Fat; 20 g Carb; 6 g Fiber; 10 g Sugar; 139 mg Calcium; 4 mg Iron; 254 mg Sodium; 736 mg Cholesterol

Poached Eggs over Bell Peppers and Spinach

Yield: 1 serving

2 to 3 eggs
1   teaspoon olive oil
3   ounces onion, thinly sliced (about 1/2 medium onion)
1   garlic clove, minced
3   ounces red bell peppers, seeded, ribs removed, and thinly sliced
    (about 1/2 medium bell pepper)
3   ounces fresh spinach, thinly sliced
1   pinch nutmeg
Salt and pepper to taste

Grease an elongated casserole with olive oil and set aside.

Heat the oil in a nonstick pan over medium heat. Add the onion and sauté until translucent. Add the garlic, bell peppers, and cook for 2 minutes. Add the spinach, nutmeg, and season to taste.

Meanwhile, bring a pan filled with water to boil. Reduce the heat under the boiling water to a point where the water barely bubbles. Break the eggs and slide them one by one into the simmering water. Make sure the eggs do not touch.

Spread the vegetables on the casserole. Using a slotted spoon carefully transfer the eggs to the prepared casserole, sprinkle pepper, and serve immediately.

Per Serving (2 eggs): 309 Cal (47% from Fat, 25% from Protein, 28% from Carb); 20 g Protein; 17 g Tot Fat; 4 g Sat Fat; 8 g Mono Fat; 22 g Carb; 5 g Fiber; 9 g Sugar; 196 mg Calcium; 5 mg Iron; 236 mg Sodium; 491 mg Cholesterol
Per Serving (3 eggs): 394 Cal (50% from Fat, 27% from Protein, 23% from Carb); 27 g Protein; 23 g Tot Fat; 6 g Sat Fat; 10 g Mono Fat; 23 g Carb; 5 g Fiber; 9 g Sugar; 227 mg Calcium; 6 mg Iron; 318 mg Sodium; 736 mg Cholesterol

Cottage Cheese and Fruits

Yield: 1 serving

1/2 cup cottage cheese
1/4 cup pineapple, diced
1/4 cup nectarine, diced
1/4 cup berries
1 teaspoon flaxseeds

M ix the cottage cheese with the flaxseeds. Add in the fruits and refrigerate to chill before use.

Option: Add 1 scoop protein powder which adds 100 calories

Per Serving: 167 Cal (19% from Fat, 40% from Protein, 41% from Carb); 17 g Protein; 4 g Tot Fat; 2 g Sat Fat; 1 g Mono Fat; 17 g Carb; 4 g Fiber; 8 g Sugar; 99 mg Calcium; 1 mg Iron; 461 mg Sodium; 9 mg Cholesterol

Bell Peppers and Turkey Roll

Yield: 1 serving

3 ounces yellow squash, cut into strips (about 1/2 squash)
3 ounces bell peppers, seeded, ribs removed, and cut into strips
   (about 1/2 bell pepper)
1 tablespoon sun-dried tomatoes, minced
3 to 4 ounces turkey slices (about 1 ounce each or 3 to 4 slices)
3 to 4 tablespoons eggplant spread
6 to 8 basil leaves
Salt and pepper to taste

M ix the sun-dried tomatoes and eggplant spread in a bowl. Lay each turkey slice on a large cutting board. Spread 1 tablespoon of the prepared mixture and 2 basil leaves over each turkey slice. Divide the bell peppers and zucchini strips equally and season to taste. Roll up each turkey slice and serve immediately.

Per Serving (3 turkey slices): 180 Cal (31% from Fat, 34% from Protein, 34% from Carb); 17 g Protein; 7 g Tot Fat; 1 g Sat Fat; 1 g Mono Fat; 17 g Carb; 3 g Fiber; 7 g Sugar; 32 mg Calcium; 2 mg Iron; 1210 mg Sodium; 35 mg Cholesterol
Per Serving (4 turkey slices): 224 Cal (32% from Fat, 36% from Protein, 32% from Carb); 22 g Protein; 9 g Tot Fat; 1 g Sat Fat; 1 g Mono Fat; 19 g Carb; 3 g Fiber; 8 g Sugar; 35 mg Calcium; 2 mg Iron; 1604 mg Sodium; 46 mg Cholesterol

Chicken and Vegetables Roll

Yield: 1 serving

3 to 4 ounces zucchini, cut into strips (about 1/2 zucchini)
3 to 4 ounces red bell peppers, seeded, ribs removed, and cut
  into strips (about 1/2 bell pepper)
3 to 4 ounces chicken breast slices (about 1 ounce each or 3 to 4 slices)
3 to 4 tablespoons tapenade
Salt and pepper to taste

Lay each chicken slice on a large cutting board. Spread 1 tablespoon of tapenade over each chicken slice. Divide the zucchini and bell pepper strips equally among the chicken slice. Season to taste, roll and serve immediately or refrigerate until needed.

Per Serving (3 chicken slices): 225 Cal (49% from Fat, 28% from Protein, 23% from Carb); 16 g Protein; 13 g Tot Fat; 2 g Sat Fat; 0 g Mono Fat; 13 g Carb; 2 g Fiber; 5 g Sugar; 26 mg Calcium; 1 mg Iron; 1325 mg Sodium; 31 mg Cholesterol
Per Serving (4 chicken slices): 299 Cal (49% from Fat, 28% from Protein, 23% from Carb); 21 g Protein; 17 g Tot Fat; 2 g Sat Fat; 0 g Mono Fat; 18 g Carb; 3 g Fiber; 7 g Sugar; 34 mg Calcium; 1 mg Iron; 1766 mg Sodium; 41 mg Cholesterol

Smoked Salmon Roll

Yield: 1 serving

3 to 4 ounces smoked salmon (about 4 to 5 ½ slices)
12 to 16 asparagus, trimmed (about 12 ounces to 1 pound asparagus)
4 to 5 ½ tablespoons Boursin Light Cheese
Pepper to taste

Preheat a steamer over high heat. Add the asparagus, reduce heat, and cook until desired doneness. Remove from the steamer and blanch in ice cold water to stop the cooking process.
   Lay each smoked salmon slice on a large cutting board. Spread 1 tablespoon of Boursin over each slice. Add 3 asparagus per slice, sprinkle pepper to taste, and roll over. For the half salmon slice use one asparagus. Serve immediately or refrigerate until needed.

Per Serving: 264 Cal (33% from Fat, 45% from Protein, 22% from Carb); 31 g Protein; 10 g Tot Fat; 5 g Sat Fat; 2 g Mono Fat; 15 g Carb; 7 g Fiber; 6 g Sugar; 91 mg Calcium; 8 mg Iron; 986 mg Sodium; 32 mg Cholesterol

Fish/Seafood Entrees

A healthy diet should include plenty of fish and some shellfish, good sources of protein, fats, vitamins, and minerals, as well as many essential amino acids. In addition, one of the best sources for Omega-3 are oily fish like cod, tuna, salmon, sardines, herring, mackerel, trout, and anchovies—which are all easier to digest than meat.

You may have already heard about the health benefits of Omega-3 fatty acids, which help promote weight loss while still having a positive effect on the metabolizing of muscle proteins. Keep in mind that the protein levels of shellfish are usually a little lower than fish and, from a nutrition standpoint, can result in higher cholesterol. So be sure not to indulge on shellfish. Cooking fish and shellfish requires particular attention, as the flesh tends to be rather delicate. It is recommended that you use healthier cooking techniques such as steaming, baking, broiling, barbecuing, or sautéing in a nonstick pan with very little oil.

Shrimp with Basil and Garlic

Yield: 2 servings

- 2 tablespoons olive oil
- 6 to 8 ounces shrimps, shelled and deveined
- 1 cup onions, sliced (about 1 large onion)
- 1 cup bell peppers, seeded, ribs removed, and sliced (about 2 medium bell peppers)
- 2 large garlic cloves, minced
- 1/2 lemon, juiced
- 2 tablespoons fresh basil, minced
- 4 to 6 ounces whole wheat pasta
- Salt and pepper to taste

Cook the pasta according to package directions.

Heat 1 tablespoon of oil and the garlic in a large pan over medium heat. Add the shrimp and cook for 1 minute stirring occasionally. In another pan, heat the remaining oil. Add the onion and sauté until translucent. Add the bell pepper and sauté for another couple of minutes. Combine the lemon juice, basil, shrimp and pasta. Season to taste. Mix and continue to sauté for 1 to 2 minutes. Serve immediately.

Per Serving (3 ounces shrimp and 4 ounces cooked pasta): 483 Cal (29% from Fat, 22% from Protein, 49% from Carb); 28 g Protein; 16 g Tot Fat; 2 g Sat Fat; 10 g Mono Fat; 63 g Carb; 4 g Fiber; 5 g Sugar; 138 mg Calcium; 5 mg Iron; 139 mg Sodium; 129 mg Cholesterol
Per Serving (4 ounces shrimp and 6 ounces cooked pasta): 611 Cal (24% from Fat, 24% from Protein, 52% from Carb); 38 g Protein; 17 g Tot Fat; 2 g Sat Fat; 10 g Mono Fat; 84 g Carb; 4 g Fiber; 5 g Sugar; 164 mg Calcium; 7 mg Iron; 183 mg Sodium; 172 mg Cholesterol

Spicy Tuna with Avocado Spread

Yield: 2 servings

- 2 teaspoons olive oil
- Two 3 to 4-ounce tuna fillets
- 4 ounces red onions, diced (about 1/2 large onion)
- 1 large Roma tomato, peeled and diced
- 6 ounces yellow bell peppers, seeded, ribs removed, and diced (about 1 medium bell pepper)
- 1 jalapeno, seeded and diced
- 1/2 avocado, puréed
- 2 tablespoons low-fat yogurt
- 1 tablespoon cilantro
- 1/4 lime, juiced
- Tabasco
- Cajun spices
- Salt to taste

Mix the avocado with the lime juice. Mix in the yogurt, jalapeno chiles, cilantro, and season to taste. Add tabasco to taste and refrigerate until needed.

Preheat the broiler. Sprinkle Cajun spices on both sides of the fillets. Place the fillets on a greased baking sheet and broil for 2 to 3 minutes. Turnover and continue to cook for 3 to 4 minutes or until the fish flesh starts to flake. You may slightly salt before serving.

Meanwhile, heat the remaining oil in a large pan over medium heat. Add the onion and sauté until translucent. Add the yellow bell peppers and continue to sauté for 2 minutes. Mix in the tomatoes and cook for 2 more minutes. Add a little Cajun spices and lightly salt.

Plate the vegetables, top with the tuna, avocado spread, and serve immediately.

Per Serving (3 ounces tuna fillet): 279 Cal (40% from Fat, 32% from Protein, 27% from Carb); 24 g Protein; 13 g Tot Fat; 2 g Sat Fat; 8 g Mono Fat; 20 g Carb; 6 g Fiber; 6 g Sugar; 71 mg Calcium; 2 mg Iron; 51 mg Sodium; 40 mg Cholesterol
Per Serving (4 ounces tuna fillet): 309 Cal (37% from Fat, 38% from Protein, 25% from Carb); 30 g Protein; 13 g Tot Fat; 2 g Sat Fat; 8 g Mono Fat; 20 g Carb; 6 g Fiber; 6 g Sugar; 75 mg Calcium; 2 mg Iron; 61 mg Sodium; 53 mg Cholesterol

Sea Scallops with Mandarin Wedges

Yield: 2 servings

2 teaspoons grapeseed oil
6 to 8 ounces sea scallops
2 scallions, chopped
1/2 cup fresh squeezed orange juice
1 teaspoon orange zest

1 mandarin, wedged
1/2 teaspoon rosemary, minced
4 ounces baby carrots
12 ounces zucchini (about 2 medium zucchini)
Salt and pepper to taste

Pat dry the sea scallops and sprinkle a little pepper on both sides.
Preheat a steamer over high heat. Add the carrots and cook until barely tender. Add the zucchini and steam for a minute.

Meanwhile, heat the oil in a large nonstick pan over medium heat. Add the scallops and cook until golden brown, about a minute or so. Turn and continue to cook for 1 to 2 minutes or until cooked through. Do not overcook as the scallops will become tough. Transfer the scallops to a serving platter and cover with aluminum foil to keep warm. Add the scallions and sauté quickly. Add the orange juice, orange zest, rosemary, and bring to a boil. Reduce by half; add the mandarin wedges, parsley, and sauté quickly. Pour over the sea scallops and serve immediately with the steamed carrots and zucchini.

Per Serving (3 ounces sea scallops): 221 Cal (23% from Fat, 31% from Protein, 46% from Carb); 18 g Protein; 6 g Tot Fat; 1 g Sat Fat; 1 g Mono Fat; 27 g Carb; 5 g Fiber; 15 g Sugar; 93 mg Calcium; 2 mg Iron; 198 mg Sodium; 28 mg Cholesterol
Per Serving (4 ounces sea scallops): 246 Cal (22% from Fat, 36% from Protein, 43% from Carb); 23 g Protein; 6 g Tot Fat; 1 g Sat Fat; 1 g Mono Fat; 27 g Carb; 5 g Fiber; 15 g Sugar; 100 mg Calcium; 2 mg Iron; 243 mg Sodium; 37 mg Cholesterol

Broiled Salmon with Pesto

Yield: 2 servings

2 tablespoons olive oil
4 tablespoons basil
2 tablespoons almonds
1 large garlic clove
1 teaspoon fresh thyme
1 teaspoon lemon zest
1 teaspoon lemon juice

Two 3 to 4-ounces salmon fillets
1 cup broccoli
1 cup cherry tomatoes
2 tablespoons Italian breadcrumbs
1/2 lemon cut into 2 wedges
Salt and pepper to taste

In a food processor puree the basil, almonds, garlic, thyme, lemon zest, lemon juice, and olive oil. Season to taste and set aside.

Preheat the oven to 400° F. Spread the pesto over the salmon fillets and top with Italian breadcrumbs. Grease a baking sheet and add the fillets. Bake for 7 to 8 minutes or until the flesh starts to flake. Time may vary based on the thickness of the fish.

Meanwhile preheat a steamer over high heat. Turn the broiler on and brown the fish breadcrumbs until golden brown, about 2 minutes. Steam the broccoli for 1 minute. Add the tomatoes and continue to steam for 1 minute. Serve the fillets with the broccoli, tomatoes, and lemon wedges.

Per Serving (3 ounces salmon fillet): 360 Cal (53% from Fat, 25% from Protein, 22% from Carb); 24 g Protein; 22 g Tot Fat; 3 g Sat Fat; 14 g Mono Fat; 21 g Carb; 5 g Fiber; 4 g Sugar; 328 mg Calcium; 3 mg Iron; 136 mg Sodium; 33 mg Cholesterol
Per Serving (4 ounces salmon fillet): 400 Cal (51% from Fat, 29% from Protein, 20% from Carb); 30 g Protein; 24 g Tot Fat; 4 g Sat Fat; 14 g Mono Fat; 21 g Carb; 5 g Fiber; 4 g Sugar; 398 mg Calcium; 3 mg Iron; 157 mg Sodium; 44 mg Cholesterol

Steamed Salmon with Fennel

Yield: 2 servings

Two 3 to 4-ounce salmon fillets
2 ounces leeks, white part only and julienned (about 1/2 leek)
2 ounces carrots, julienned (about 1/2 small carrot)
12 ounces fennel bulbs, julienned (about 1 large bulb)
1 garlic clove, minced
2 tablespoons Pastis or anisette (You may substitute vegetable stock)
2 pinches Herbs de Provence
1 teaspoon fennel seeds
Salt and pepper to taste

Preheat the oven to 400° F.
   Prepare two aluminum foil packets. Place the vegetables in the center of the foil, spread the fennel seeds, and season to taste. Top with the seasoned fish and sprinkle the Herbs de Provence. Fold the aluminum foil a bit; add the Pastis, and close tightly. Place on a baking dish and bake for 10 to 12 minutes or until the salmon starts to flake. Transfer each foil to a serving plate, open carefully, and serve immediately.

> **Per Serving (3 ounces salmon fillet):** 233 Cal (20% from Fat, 37% from Protein, 42% from Carb); 22 g Protein; 5 g Tot Fat; 1 g Sat Fat; 2 g Mono Fat; 25 g Carb; 7 g Fiber; 3 g Sugar; 360 mg Calcium; 3 mg Iron; 273 mg Sodium; 33 mg Cholesterol
> **Per Serving (4 ounces salmon fillet):** 273 Cal (23% from Fat, 41% from Protein, 37% from Carb); 28 g Protein; 7 g Tot Fat; 2 g Sat Fat; 2 g Mono Fat; 25 g Carb; 7 g Fiber; 3 g Sugar; 430 mg Calcium; 3 mg Iron; 294 mg Sodium; 44 mg Cholesterol

Cod Fish with Jicama & Red Bell Pepper Slaw

Yield: 2 servings

1 teaspoon olive oil
Two 3 to 4-ounce cod fillets
6 ounces Jicama, julienned (about 1 medium Jicama)
6 ounces red bell peppers, seeded, ribs removed and julienned (about 1 medium red bell pepper)
4 ounces carrots, julienned (about 1 small carrot)
1 green onion, julienned
2 tablespoons olive oil
2 tablespoons lime juice
2 tablespoon fresh parsley, minced
3 pinches ground cumin
Salt and pepper to taste

Place the julienned Jicama, red bell peppers, carrots, and green onions in a bowl. Whisk 2 tablespoons olive oil, lime juice, parsley, and two pinches ground cumin. Add the dressing to the vegetables, season to taste, mix well, and set aside.
   Sprinkle pepper and ground cumin over both sides of the fish. Heat 1 teaspoon olive oil in nonstick pan over medium heat. Add the fish and sauté until golden brown, about 2 minutes. Turnover and continue to cook until the fish starts to flake.
   Meanwhile, quickly sauté the prepared slaw in a nonstick pan over medium heat. Lightly season the cod fillets with salt, if desired.
   Transfer the slaw to two serving plates, top with the cod fillets, and serve immediately.

> **Per Serving (3 ounces cod fillet):** 297 Cal (50% from Fat, 23% from Protein, 27% from Carb); 18 g Protein; 17 g Tot Fat; 2 g Sat Fat; 12 g Mono Fat; 21 g Carb; 8 g Fiber; 8 g Sugar; 65 mg Calcium; 2 mg Iron; 95 mg Sodium; 37 mg Cholesterol
> **Per Serving (4 ounces cod fillet):** 320 Cal (47% from Fat, 28% from Protein, 25% from Carb); 23 g Protein; 17 g Tot Fat; 2 g Sat Fat; 12 g Mono Fat; 21 g Carb; 8 g Fiber; 8 g Sugar; 70 mg Calcium; 2 mg Iron; 110 mg Sodium; 49 mg Cholesterol

Jamaican Red Snapper

Yield: 2 servings

Two 3 to 4-ounce red snapper fillets
5   ounces carrots cut into thin diagonal
    slices (about 1 medium carrot)
5   ounces yellow squash cut into thin diago-
    nal slices (about 1 medium squash)
6   ounces pea pods
1   large garlic clove, minced

1   tablespoon fresh ginger, minced
1   teaspoon low-sodium soy sauce
2   tablespoons chives, chopped
2   teaspoons sesame oil
Jamaican jerk spices or rub
Salt and pepper to taste

Preheat a pan with water. Parboil each vegetable (carrots, squash, and pea pods) separately and until barely tender. Blanch immediately in ice cold water to stop the cooking process.

Preheat the broiler with the rack five inches away from the broiler. Spread the spices over the fillets and place them on a greased cookie sheet. Broil for a few minutes or until the fillets starts to flake. Time may vary based on thickness.

Meanwhile, heat the oil in a large nonstick pan over medium heat. Sauté the ginger and garlic quickly. Add the vegetables and sauté for another minute. Add the soy sauce, chives, and season with pepper. Bring to a boil and serve immediately with the red snapper fillets.

Per Serving (3 ounces red snapper fillet): 227 Cal (24% from Fat, 39% from Protein, 37% from Carb); 23 g Protein; 6 g Tot Fat; 1 g Sat Fat; 2 g Mono Fat; 21 g Carb; 6 g Fiber; 8 g Sugar; 127 mg Calcium; 3 mg Iron; 263 mg Sodium; 31 mg Cholesterol
Per Serving (4 ounces red snapper fillet): 255 Cal (23% from Fat, 44% from Protein, 33% from Carb); 28 g Protein; 7 g Tot Fat; 1 g Sat Fat; 2 g Mono Fat; 21 g Carb; 6 g Fiber; 8 g Sugar; 136 mg Calcium; 3 mg Iron; 281 mg Sodium; 42 mg Cholesterol

Ahi Tartar

Yield: 2 servings

Two 3 to 4-ounce Ahi fillets
2   tablespoons shallots, chopped
4   ounces cucumbers (about 1/3
    large cucumber)
1   lemon
1   lime
3   ounces red bell peppers, seeded and ribs
    removed, diced (about1/2 medium
    red bell pepper)

1   jalapeno chile, seeded and diced
1   sage leaf
2   tablespoons basil, chopped
1/2 teaspoon green tea
1/2 teaspoon honey
2   tablespoons olive oil
1   cup baby lettuce mix
Salt and pepper to taste

Take nice strips of the lemon and lime zests. Mince and set aside. Juice the lemon, lime, and set aside. Cut the cucumber in half and remove seeds. Cut into half again and dice. Warm up on low heat the lemon juice, lime juice, tea powder, and sage until the honey is well incorporated. Remove and cool down. Refrigerate to get cold.

Dice the Ahi, place it into a soup plate and season to taste. Mix in the shallot, cucumber, red bell pepper, jalapeno chiles, and basil. Drizzle half of the olive oil, add the cold marinade, and refrigerate for 20 to 30 minutes.

Equally divide the baby greens among two ice cold plates. With a slotted spoon, scoop out the Ahi Tartar. Drizzle a little bit of the marinade, the remaining olive oil, and serve immediately.

Per Serving (3 ounces Ahi): 298 Cal (51% from Fat, 28% from Protein, 21% from Carb); 22 g Protein; 18 g Tot Fat; 3 g Sat Fat; 11 g Mono Fat; 17 g Carb; 5 g Fiber; 5 g Sugar; 74 mg Calcium; 2 mg Iron; 42 mg Sodium; 32 mg Cholesterol
Per Serving (4 ounces Ahi): 339 Cal (49% from Fat, 32% from Protein, 19% from Carb); 29 g Protein; 20 g Tot Fat; 3 g Sat Fat; 12 g Mono Fat; 17 g Carb; 5 g Fiber; 5 g Sugar; 76 mg Calcium; 2 mg Iron; 53 mg Sodium; 43 mg Cholesterol

Meat / Poultry Entrees

It is important to your health that you choose a good source of protein and make sure you get the right amount. You may already know that animal protein is not as healthy for you as the protein from fresh fruits and vegetables; this is because meat can raise cholesterol levels. To minimize cholesterol, look for lean protein sources. Additionally, seek out organic meat. This is healthier for you, due to the animal's natural diet.

Here are some good general rules for selecting meat: choose venison or ostrich over beef, and choose white meat such as chicken or turkey breast over darker meat. Note that lamb and pork, which are higher in fat, should be eaten sparingly, (this is why you will find only one recipe for each in this section.) When you do eat pork, choose pork loin tender cuts and employ healthy cooking techniques, such as those described on the following pages, which will limit the addition of fat and calories during preparation while also preserving the succulent flavor of the meat.

Chicken Burgers with Lettuce Wraps

Yield: 2 servings

Two 3 to 4-ounce chicken burgers
2 garlic cloves, minced
2 tablespoons low-cal Caesar dressing
1 white anchovy fillet

8 lettuce leaves
2 tablespoons Parmesan Cheese
Canola oil
Salt and pepper to taste

In a food processor, puree the anchovy fillet with the dressing. Add a little water to thin out. Lightly season the burgers and shape them to fit in the lettuce leaves. Do not allow the meat to touch the leaves. Heat up 2 tablespoons olive oil with the minced garlic. Remove at the first boil and set aside.

Preheat the grill on medium high heat. Don't forget to grease the grill before adding the burgers. Cook them for 3 to 5 minutes on each side or until cooked through. Meanwhile, carefully brush the garlic oil over the lettuce leaves.

Place two leaves on a plate, top with one burger, spread 1 tablespoon Caesar dressing, sprinkle cheese and fold a bit over the top. Top with 2 more leaves and tuck underneath to seal. Serve immediately with your favorite accompaniment. You may use toothpick to hold for presentation.

Suggestion: Serve with Eggplant Mediterranean

Per Serving (3 ounces chicken burger): 334 Cal (52% from Fat, 37% from Protein, 11% from Carb); 31 g Protein; 19 g Tot Fat; 4 g Sat Fat; 12 g Mono Fat; 9 g Carb; 1 g Fiber; 3 g Sugar; 131 mg Calcium; 2 mg Iron; 408 mg Sodium; 80 mg Cholesterol
Per Serving (4 ounces chicken burger): 381 Cal (49% from Fat, 42% from Protein, 9% from Carb); 40 g Protein; 20 g Tot Fat; 4 g Sat Fat; 12 g Mono Fat; 9 g Carb; 1 g Fiber; 3 g Sugar; 135 mg Calcium; 2 mg Iron; 429 mg Sodium; 104 mg Cholesterol

Lamb Chops with Garlic Spread

Yield: 2 servings

3 teaspoons olive oil
Two 3 to 4-ounce loin lamb chops
1 tablespoon minced garlic
1 teaspoon parsley
1 teaspoon minced rosemary
1/4 teaspoon dry crushed red pepper
2 cups green beans
Salt and pepper to taste

Bring to a boil enough water to cover the green beans. Add 1 teaspoon of salt, the green beans, and bring to boil. Reduce heat and simmer until tender. Drain and transfer to a serving bowl. Add 1 teaspoon olive oil, season to taste, and mix well.

Mix 1 teaspoon olive oil, garlic, parsley, rosemary, and dry crushed red pepper in a bowl. Rub the garlic spread over the lamb chops.

Heat the remaining olive oil in a nonstick pan over medium heat. Add the lamb chops and cook for 3 to 4 minutes on each side or until desired. Serve immediately with the prepared green beans.

Per Serving (3 ounces lamb chops): 213 Cal (46% from Fat, 36% from Protein, 17% from Carb); 20 g Protein; 11 g Tot Fat; 3 g Sat Fat; 7 g Mono Fat; 9 g Carb; 4 g Fiber; 2 g Sugar; 58 mg Calcium; 3 mg Iron; 62 mg Sodium; 54 mg Cholesterol
Per Serving (4 ounces lamb chops): 250 Cal (45% from Fat, 40% from Protein, 15% from Carb); 25 g Protein; 12 g Tot Fat; 3 g Sat Fat; 7 g Mono Fat; 9 g Carb; 4 g Fiber; 2 g Sugar; 60 mg Calcium; 4 mg Iron; 81 mg Sodium; 73 mg Cholesterol

New York Steaks with Mushrooms and Onions

Yield: 2 servings

Two 3 to 4-ounce New York steaks
2 teaspoons olive oil
8 ounces onions, sliced (about 1 large onion)
8 ounces mushrooms, sliced
1 garlic clove, minced
1 tablespoon parsley, minced
2 tablespoons Dijon mustard
Salt and pepper to taste

Preheat the broiler. Brush a little olive oil over the steaks and season with pepper. Broil for 3 to 5 minutes on each side or until desired. Sprinkle a little salt before serving.

Meanwhile, heat 1 teaspoon olive oil in a nonstick pan over medium heat. Add the onions and slightly brown. Add the mushrooms, garlic, and continue to cook until the mushrooms are barely tender. Add the parsley and season to taste.

Plate the vegetables in the center of a serving platter and top with the steaks. Serve with Dijon mustard on the side.

Per Serving (3 ounces New York Steak): 340 Cal (42% from Fat, 34% from Protein, 24% from Carb); 29 g Protein; 16 g Tot Fat; 5 g Sat Fat; 8 g Mono Fat; 21 g Carb; 4 g Fiber; 8 g Sugar; 88 mg Calcium; 3 mg Iron; 235 mg Sodium; 57 mg Cholesterol
Per Serving (4 ounces New York Steak): 405 Cal (44% from Fat, 36% from Protein, 21% from Carb); 37 g Protein; 20 g Tot Fat; 6 g Sat Fat; 10 g Mono Fat; 21 g Carb; 4 g Fiber; 8 g Sugar; 94 mg Calcium; 3 mg Iron; 251 mg Sodium; 76 mg Cholesterol

Chicken Breasts with Tomato Sauce

Yield: 2 servings

1 teaspoon olive oil
Two 3 to 4-ounce chicken breasts
4 small Roma tomatoes (about 1 pound)
3/4 cup pearl onions

1/4 cup dry white wine
1 pinch Italian herbs
1 tablespoon fresh basil, minced
Salt and pepper to taste

Par-boil the pearl onions for a couple of minutes. Remove the pearl onions from the water and let cool. Peel them and set aside.

Make a small X incision into the tops of the tomatoes. Heat some water over high heat and bring to boil. Blanch the tomatoes for 15 to 20 seconds. Remove and place in ice-cold water to stop the cooking process. Peel, seed, and dice the tomatoes.

Heat the oil in a large saucepan. Add the chicken and sauté until golden brown. Turnover and continue to cook for 2 minutes. Deglaze the pan with the wine and reduce a little. Add the tomatoes, pearl onions, Italian herbs, and season to taste. Reduce heat and cook for 10 minutes or until the chicken is cooked through. Add the basil and cook for another minute. Transfer to a serving platter and serve immediately.

Suggestion: Serve with wild rice and mushrooms

Per Serving (3 ounces chicken breast): 211 Cal (18% from Fat, 46% from Protein, 36% from Carb); 23 g Protein; 4 g Tot Fat; 1 g Sat Fat; 2 g Mono Fat; 17 g Carb; 4 g Fiber; 10 g Sugar; 64 mg Calcium; 2 mg Iron; 71 mg Sodium; 49 mg Cholesterol
Per Serving (4 ounces chicken breast): 242 Cal (17% from Fat, 52% from Protein, 31% from Carb); 29 g Protein; 4 g Tot Fat; 1 g Sat Fat; 2 g Mono Fat; 17 g Carb; 4 g Fiber; 10 g Sugar; 67 mg Calcium; 2 mg Iron; 89 mg Sodium; 66 mg Cholesterol

Chicken Breasts with Spinach and Pepper Jack

Yield: 2 servings

1   teaspoon olive oil
Two 3 to 4-ounce chicken breasts
2   pepper jack cheese slices
8   spinach leaves, cleaned and pat dry
1   shallot, minced
1/4 cup chicken stock

Italian herbs
2   cups fresh spinach, cleaned and pat dry
1   lemon
Salt and pepper to taste
Twine

Place the chicken breasts between two plastic wrap sheets. Flatten with a mallet until fairly thin. Sprinkle pepper and Italian herbs. Add one slice of pepper jack cheese and the spinach leaves. Roll tightly making sure the cheese has no way out and secure with twine.

Heat the oil in a sauté pan over high heat. Add the chicken rolls, placing the folded side down first. Brown and turn over. Once browned, add the shallot, stock, a teaspoon lemon juice, a pinch of Italian herbs, and bring to boil. Reduce heat, cover, and continue to cook for 10 minutes.

Meanwhile, preheat a steamer. Add the spinach and cook for a minute or until barely wilted. Serve immediately with the chicken rolls and lemon wedges.

Per Serving (3 ounces chicken breast): 265 Cal (42% from Fat, 41% from Protein, 17% from Carb); 29 g Protein; 13 g Tot Fat; 6 g Sat Fat; 5 g Mono Fat; 12 g Carb; 4 g Fiber; 1 g Sugar; 288 mg Calcium; 3 mg Iron; 368 mg Sodium; 76 mg Cholesterol
Per Serving (4 ounces chicken breast): 297 Cal (39% from Fat, 46% from Protein, 15% from Carb); 35 g Protein; 13 g Tot Fat; 6 g Sat Fat; 5 g Mono Fat; 12 g Carb; 4 g Fiber; 1 g Sugar; 291 mg Calcium; 3 mg Iron; 386 mg Sodium; 93 mg Cholesterol

Roasted Cornish Hen with Chinese Five Spices Blend

Yield: 2 servings

1 Cornish hen
1 teaspoon sesame oil
1 tablespoon honey
1 teaspoon Oriental hot mustard
1 teaspoon ginger, minced
1 teaspoon garlic, minced
1 teaspoon Chinese Five Spices Blend
Salt and pepper to taste

Preheat the oven to 350°F.
Wash and pat dry the hen. Combine the honey, mustard, ginger, garlic, and spices. Brush the mixture over the hen. Roast for an hour or until the juices come out clear. Time may vary based on the hen size. Cut the hen in half and transfer to a serving platter. Drizzle sesame oil and serve immediately.

Suggestion: Serve with Snap Peas with Garlic

Per Serving (1/2 Cornish hen): 393 Cal (60% from Fat, 30% from Protein, 10% from Carb); 29 g Protein; 26 g Tot Fat; 7 g Sat Fat; 11 g Mono Fat; 9 g Carb; 0 g Fiber; 9 g Sugar; 23 mg Calcium; 1 mg Iron; 103 mg Sodium; 170 mg Cholesterol

Venison with Spicy Raspberry Sauce

Yield: 2 servings

2 teaspoons grapeseed oil
Two 3 to 4-ounce venison steaks
1 small shallot, minced
1/4 to 1/2 teaspoon black peppercorns,
   crushed (based on how spicy you like)
1 pinch dry thyme
2 tablespoons aged balsamic vinegar

1/2 cup Cabernet Sauvignon
1/2 cup raspberries
2 tablespoons demi-glace (if not available,
   substitute brown sauce)
1 tablespoon freshly minced parsley
Salt and pepper to taste

Puree half the raspberries in a food processor. Pass through a sieve and set aside.
   Heat the oil in a nonstick pan over medium-high heat. Add the venison steaks and sauté until golden brown. Turnover and continue to cook for 2 to 3 minutes. Transfer the steaks to a plate and cover with aluminum foil to keep warm. Add the shallots, peppercorns, thyme, vinegar, wine, raspberry sauce, and deglaze the pan. Bring to a boil and reduce liquid by half. Add demi-glace, steaks juices, season to taste, and bring to a boil. Add the steaks, remaining raspberries, and continue to simmer for a minute. Serve immediately.

Serve with Green Beans and Almonds

Per Serving (3 ounces venison loin): 216 Cal (35% from Fat, 47% from Protein, 19% from Carb); 21 g Protein; 7 g Tot Fat; 1 g Sat Fat; 1 g Mono Fat; 8 g Carb; 2 g Fiber; 2 g Sugar; 28 mg Calcium; 4 mg Iron; 99 mg Sodium; 72 mg Cholesterol
Per Serving (4 ounces venison loin): 250 Cal (32% from Fat, 52% from Protein, 16% from Carb); 27 g Protein; 8 g Tot Fat; 2 g Sat Fat; 2 g Mono Fat; 8 g Carb; 2 g Fiber; 2 g Sugar; 29 mg Calcium; 5 mg Iron; 113 mg Sodium; 96 mg Cholesterol

Turkey Breast with Italian Herbs

Yield: 8 to 10 servings

1 tablespoon olive oil
2 pounds turkey breast (with skin)
4 teaspoons Italian herbs
A bunch of fresh basil leaves
1/4 cup chicken stock
Salt and pepper to taste

Preheat the oven to 350° F.
   Mix 1 tablespoon of Italian herbs with a little pepper. Spread all over the turkey breast under its skin. Add as many basil leaves as you can fit under the skin without breaking it. Brush olive oil over the skin.
   Place the turkey breast skin side up in a roasting pan. Pour 1/4 cup of chicken stock in the pan, add the remaining Italian herbs, and bake for an hour or until a meat thermometer registers 180° F. Keep moistening with chicken stock. Do not allow the pan to get dry in order to keep the turkey breast moist. Transfer the turkey breast to a platter and let cool before slicing.

Great way to prepare your own turkey breast meat for salads, sandwiches, rolls, etc....

Per Serving (10 servings of 3 ounces): 159 Cal (46% from Fat, 52% from Protein, 2% from Carb); 20 g Protein; 8 g Tot Fat; 2 g Sat Fat; 3 g Mono Fat; 1 g Carb; 0 g Fiber; 0 g Sugar; 21 mg Calcium; 2 mg Iron; 95 mg Sodium; 59 mg Cholesterol
Per Serving (8 servings of 4 ounces): 199 Cal (46% from Fat, 52% from Protein, 2% from Carb); 25 g Protein; 10 g Tot Fat; 2 g Sat Fat; 4 g Mono Fat; 1 g Carb; 0 g Fiber; 0 g Sugar; 26 mg Calcium; 2 mg Iron; 119 mg Sodium; 74 mg Cholesterol

Pork Loin with Figs

Yield: 2 servings

8 to 10 ounces pork loin	1/2 cup veal stock
1 teaspoon olive oil	1 fresh rosemary branch
4 figs	1 acorn squash, halved and seeded
1/2 orange	2 teaspoons sliced almonds
1/4 cup Chardonnay wine	Salt and pepper to taste
1 tablespoon honey	

Preheat the broiler. Cover a baking sheet with parchment paper. Spread over the almonds and brown under the broiler. Remove from the pan and set aside for later use.

Preheat the oven to 350° F.

Place the loin in a roasting pan, rub with a little oil, and sprinkle pepper. Bake until the inside temperature reaches 185° F.

Make an X incision into the top of the figs. Place the figs and the acorn squash (cut side down) into a baking pan. Bring to a boil the orange juice, wine, and honey in a saucepan over high heat. Mix well and pour over the figs and acorn squash. Bake for 30 minutes at 350° F spooning the sauce over every 10 minutes.

Remove the roast from the pan and set aside in a plate. Sprinkle salt to taste. Cover with aluminum foil to keep warm. Allow 10 to 15 minutes before slicing.

Deglaze the pan with the stock and scrape out all the particles in the bottom and side of the pan. Add the rosemary branch and pour in the sauce rendered by the acorn and figs. Bring to boil and reduce to concentrate flavors. If necessary, thicken with a little cornstarch water mixture and bring to a boil. Add the parsley, any rendered meat juices, and bring to a boil. Adjust seasonings and pour over the loin. Serve immediately with the figs and acorn squash.

Per Serving (3 ounces pork loin): 434 Cal (16% from Fat, 26% from Protein, 58% from Carb); 29 g Protein; 8 g Tot Fat; 2 g Sat Fat; 4 g Mono Fat; 63 g Carb; 9 g Fiber; 30 g Sugar; 165 mg Calcium; 4 mg Iron; 187 mg Sodium; 74 mg Cholesterol
Per Serving (4 ounces pork loin): 468 Cal (17% from Fat, 29% from Protein, 54% from Carb); 35 g Protein; 9 g Tot Fat; 2 g Sat Fat; 5 g Mono Fat; 63 g Carb; 9 g Fiber; 30 g Sugar; 166 mg Calcium; 5 mg Iron; 201 mg Sodium; 92 mg Cholesterol

Soups/Salads

Soups and salads are very versatile and can be served as an appetizer, main course, side dish, or even dessert. They're quick and healthy meal options, and can be a great way to use left-overs. In addition, salad recipes don't require much cooking knowledge, as the techniques used here are very basic.

Here are a few important things to keep in mind whenever you prepare soup or a salad. First, stay away from croutons in soups and avoid unhealthy salad dressings. Healthy dressing choices include oil and vinegar or citrus juice with fresh herbs, and apple cider vinegar can be beneficial to your health due to its cleansing and healing properties. Be careful not to overcook the vegetables you add to soup bases as they will lose their nutrients. This can be tricky because a soup's ingredients will continue to cook as long as the soup is hot, even after you've taken the soup off the stove. Try to undercook the vegetables to allow for that extra time and to preserve their nutritive values. Use dry herbs at first and finish with fresh herbs (using fresh herbs at the beginning will only be a waste of money, as the flavors will evaporate during the cooking process.) For balanced nutrition, be sure to include lean proteins, complex carbohydrates, and vegetables in your soups and salads.

Beans, Vegetables, and Avocado Salad

Yield: 7 to 10 servings.

4 ounces garbanzos
4 ounces black beans
4 ounces red beans
4 ounces green beans, trimmed and cut into bite sized pieces
1 ounce red onions, diced (about 1/4 small onion)
8 ounces tomatoes, diced (about 2 small tomatoes)

1 garlic clove, minced
2 tablespoons olive oil
1/4 cup white balsamic vinegar
1 ½ tablespoons freshly minced salad herbs
1 avocado, diced
Salt and pepper to taste

In a bowl mix the garlic, oil, vinegar, and herbs.
Cook the beans separately following the packages instructions. Generally, it takes about 30 to 45 minutes to cook these types of beans.

Place the green beans with a little salt in a pan and bring to a boil over high heat. Cook to desired. Strain and place immediately in ice-cold water to stop the cooking process. Strain and pat dry.

Place all the beans and red onions in a large bowl. Add the tomatoes and dressing. Season to taste and refrigerate for an hour. Before serving, add the avocado.

Per Serving (3 ounces): 184 Cal (30% from Fat, 17% from Protein, 53% from Carb); 8 g Protein; 6 g Tot Fat; 1 g Sat Fat; 4 g Mono Fat; 26 g Carb; 8 g Fiber; 3 g Sugar; 57 mg Calcium; 3 mg Iron; 10 mg Sodium; 0 mg Cholesterol
Per Serving (4 ounces): 246 Cal (30% from Fat, 17% from Protein, 53% from Carb); 11 g Protein; 9 g Tot Fat; 1 g Sat Fat; 5 g Mono Fat; 34 g Carb; 11 g Fiber; 4 g Sugar; 76 mg Calcium; 3 mg Iron; 14 mg Sodium; 0 mg Cholesterol

Beets and Chicken Salad

Yield: 2 servings

10 ounces cooked beets, trimmed and diced
4 ounces Romaine heart leaves
1/3 small onion, diced
1/4 cup walnuts
1 small apple, diced and mixed with a little lemon juice (about 4 ounces)
Two 3 to 4-ounce cooked chicken breasts, diced
2 tablespoons vinaigrette
Salt and pepper to taste

Place the beets, romaine leaves, red onion, and chicken in a large bowl. Mix in the vinaigrette and adjust seasoning. Equally divide the salad in two plates. Top with the diced apple, walnut, and serve immediately.

Option: Add 2 tablespoons feta cheese

Per Serving (3 ounces chicken breast): 311 Cal (40% from Fat, 24% from Protein, 36% from Carb); 20 g Protein; 15 g Tot Fat; 2 g Sat Fat; 2 g Mono Fat; 30 g Carb; 7 g Fiber; 18 g Sugar; 69 mg Calcium; 3 mg Iron; 1283 mg Sodium; 31 mg Cholesterol
Per Serving (4 ounces chicken breast): 334 Cal (37% from Fat, 28% from Protein, 35% from Carb); 25 g Protein; 15 g Tot Fat; 2 g Sat Fat; 2 g Mono Fat; 31 g Carb; 7 g Fiber; 19 g Sugar; 71 mg Calcium; 3 mg Iron; 1592 mg Sodium; 41 mg Cholesterol

Per Serving (feta cheese): 25 Cal (72% from Fat, 21% from Protein, 6% from Carb); 1 g Protein; 2 g Tot Fat; 1 g Sat Fat; 0 g Mono Fat; 0 g Carb; 0 g Fiber; 0 g Sugar; 46 mg Calcium; 0 mg Iron

Grapefruit and Crabmeat Salad

Yield: 2 servings

1 large pink grapefruit (about 16 ounces grapefruit)
Two 3 to 4-ounce crabmeat portions (without excess water)
2 tablespoons low-fat canola mayonnaise
1 cup lettuce, shredded
1 tablespoon freshly minced cilantro
Chili powder to taste
Salt and pepper to taste

Place the crabmeat in a bowl.
   Cut the grapefruit in half. Insert a thin knife all around the skin to loosen up the flesh. Separate the flesh from the skin and place the flesh on a cutting board. Dice the flesh small and transfer to the crabmeat bowl. Add mayonnaise, chili powder, cilantro, and season to taste. Cover with plastic wrap and refrigerate for half an hour.
   Equally divide the lettuce in two plates and top with the prepared grapefruit crabmeat salad.

Per Serving (3 ounces crabmeat): 192 Cal (19% from Fat, 37% from Protein, 43% from Carb); 18 g Protein; 4 g Tot Fat; 1 g Sat Fat; 1 g Mono Fat; 21 g Carb; 3 g Fiber; 16 g Sugar; 88 mg Calcium; 1 mg Iron; 936 mg Sodium; 48 mg Cholesterol
Per Serving (4 ounces crabmeat): 219 Cal (19% from Fat, 43% from Protein, 38% from Carb); 24 g Protein; 5 g Tot Fat; 1 g Sat Fat; 1 g Mono Fat; 21 g Carb; 3 g Fiber; 16 g Sugar; 105 mg Calcium; 1 mg Iron; 1240 mg Sodium; 63 mg Cholesterol

Salmon and Vegetables Carpaccio

Yield: 2 servings

6 to 8 ounces smoked salmon thin slices
8 ounces cucumber, peeled (about 1 medium cucumber)
8 ounces yellow squash, peeled (about 1 large yellow squash)
2 green onions, minced
2 teaspoons fresh dill, minced
4 tablespoons olive oil
1 lemon
Salt and pepper to taste

Remove a couple of zest strips from the lemon and mince. Juice the lemon and set aside in a bowl. Add the olive oil, 1 teaspoon dill, half of the prepared zest, and season to taste.
   Thinly slice the cucumber and the zucchini. Refrigerate until use.
   Equally divide the salmon in two plates, season to taste, and sprinkle dill. Pour half the dressing over and refrigerate for 20 minutes. In the center of the salmon slices and in a round formation, alternate the cucumber and zucchini slices. Season lightly and garnish with the green onions, remaining zest and dill. Pour over the remaining dressing and serve immediately.

Per Serving (3 ounces smoked salmon): 388 Cal (69% from Fat, 18% from Protein, 13% from Carb); 19 g Protein; 31 g Tot Fat; 5 g Sat Fat; 22 g Mono Fat; 14 g Carb; 5 g Fiber; 4 g Sugar; 104 mg Calcium; 3 mg Iron; 687 mg Sodium; 20 mg Cholesterol
Per Serving (4 ounces smoked salmon): 421 Cal (66% from Fat, 22% from Protein, 12% from Carb); 24 g Protein; 33 g Tot Fat; 5 g Sat Fat; 22 g Mono Fat; 14 g Carb; 5 g Fiber; 4 g Sugar; 107 mg Calcium; 3 mg Iron; 910 mg Sodium; 26 mg Cholesterol

Calamari Salad

8 to 10 ounces Calamari or squids
1   garlic clove, minced
2   tablespoons olive oil
1/2 lemon, juiced
4   ounces baby greens
6   ounces red bell peppers, chopped (about 1 medium red bell pepper)
4   ounces tomatoes, sliced (about 1 small tomato)
2   ounces red onions, sliced (about 1/2 small onion)
1   tablespoon freshly minced basil
Salt and pepper to taste

Clean and then cut the calamari into bite size pieces. Boil the calamari in water for 20 minutes or until tender. Drain and transfer to a serving bowl. Add the garlic, olive oil, lemon juice, half the basil, and season to taste. Refrigerate for a few hours to allow marinade to flavor the calamari.

Dress up four plates with lettuce and top with the marinated calamari. Equally divide the red bell pepper, tomato, red onion among the four plates. Sprinkle a little more fresh basil and serve immediately.

Option: You may substitute frozen, cleaned calamari.

Per Serving (4 ounces calamari): 298 Cal (45% from Fat, 27% from Protein, 28% from Carb); 21 g Protein; 16 g Tot Fat; 2 g Sat Fat; 10 g Mono Fat; 22 g Carb; 5 g Fiber; 5 g Sugar; 121 mg Calcium; 2 mg Iron; 76 mg Sodium; 264 mg Cholesterol
Per Serving (5 ounces calamari): 324 Cal (43% from Fat, 30% from Protein, 27% from Carb); 26 g Protein; 16 g Tot Fat; 2 g Sat Fat; 10 g Mono Fat; 23 g Carb; 5 g Fiber; 5 g Sugar; 130 mg Calcium; 3 mg Iron; 88 mg Sodium; 330 mg Cholesterol

Seared Ahi Salad

Two 3 to 4-ounce Ahi fillets, Sushi grade
4   ounces mixed greens
6   cherry tomatoes
4   ounces carrots, sliced diagonally
2   ounces daikon, sliced
2   ounces sugar snap peas
1   teaspoon sesame oil

1   teaspoon soy sauce
1   tablespoon lime juice
4   teaspoons olive oil
1   teaspoon ginger, minced
1   lime
Salt and pepper to taste

Mix the sesame oil, soy sauce, lime juice, 1 tablespoon olive oil, and ginger together in a bowl. Season with pepper.

Par-boil the carrot and sugar snap peas to desired tenderness. Transfer to an ice-cold water bath to stop the cooking process. Pat dry and set aside.

Mix the greens, carrots, daikon, and sugar snap peas in a bowl with the prepared dressing. Equally divide among two plates and refrigerate until use.

Preheat 1 teaspoon olive oil in a nonstick pan over high heat. Season the fish with pepper and light salt. Sear the fish for 2 minutes on both sides. You may sear longer, if you want the center of the fish more cooked.

Slice the fish and spread over the top of the prepared salad. Serve immediately with lime wedges.

Per Serving (3 ounces Ahi): 306 Cal (46% from Fat, 30% from Protein, 24% from Carb); 24 g Protein; 16 g Tot Fat; 3 g Sat Fat; 9 g Mono Fat; 19 g Carb; 6 g Fiber; 6 g Sugar; 68 mg Calcium; 2 mg Iron; 237 mg Sodium; 32 mg Cholesterol
Per Serving (4 ounces Ahi): 347 Cal (45% from Fat, 34% from Protein, 21% from Carb); 30 g Protein; 17 g Tot Fat; 3 g Sat Fat; 9 g Mono Fat; 19 g Carb; 6 g Fiber; 6 g Sugar; 70 mg Calcium; 3 mg Iron; 248 mg Sodium; 43 mg Cholesterol

Greek Salad

Yield: 2 servings

3 ounces mixed greens
2 ounces red onions, sliced (about 1/2 small onion)
3 ounces cucumbers, sliced (about 1/2 medium cucumber)
3 ounces red bell peppers, sliced (about 1/2 medium red bell pepper)
6 ounces tomatoes, sliced (about 1 large tomato)
4 teaspoons feta cheese crumbled
2 tablespoons black olives

6 white anchovy fillets
Two 3 to 4-ounce chicken breasts
1 tablespoon wine vinegar
2 tablespoons olive oil
1/2 tablespoon flaxseed oil
1 teaspoon garlic cloves, minced
1 tablespoon low-fat yogurt
1 teaspoon freshly minced oregano
1 tablespoon freshly minced parsley
Salt and pepper to taste

In a bowl, mix the vinegar, oils, and garlic. Blend in the yogurt. Add the oregano, parsley, and season to taste. In a large bowl, place the lettuce, red onions, cucumbers, bell peppers, and tomatoes. Add the dressing and mix well. Divide equally among two plates. Top with the olives, feta cheese, anchovy fillets, and serve immediately.

> **Per Serving (3 ounces chicken breast):** 324 Cal (57% from Fat, 26% from Protein, 17% from Carb); 21 g Protein; 21 g Tot Fat; 4 g Sat Fat; 12 g Mono Fat; 14 g Carb; 3 g Fiber; 7 g Sugar; 131 mg Calcium; 2 mg Iron; 1534 mg Sodium; 47 mg Cholesterol
> **Per Serving (4 ounces chicken breast):** 346 Cal (54% from Fat, 29% from Protein, 17% from Carb); 26 g Protein; 21 g Tot Fat; 4 g Sat Fat; 12 g Mono Fat; 15 g Carb; 3 g Fiber; 7 g Sugar; 133 mg Calcium; 2 mg Iron; 1842 mg Sodium; 57 mg Cholesterol

Fish Soup

Yield: 4 servings

1 teaspoon olive oil
5 ounces onions, diced (about 1 medium onion)
3 ounces carrots, diced (about 1 small carrot)
1 tablespoon minced garlic
4 ounces Chardonnay wine
3 pounds fish steaks and fillets

4 cups fish stock (low-sodium)
1 bouquet garni
6 ounces tomatoes (about 1 large tomato)
3 tablespoons parsley, minced
1 strip orange zest
1 teaspoon fennel seeds
Salt and pepper to taste

Make a small X incision on the top and bottom of the tomato. Blanch the tomato for 15 to 20 seconds. Remove and place the tomato in ice-cold water to stop the cooking process. Peel, seed, and dice the tomatoes. Set aside.

Heat the oil in a large pan over high heat. Add the onions and sauté until translucent. Add the carrots, garlic, and sauté for 2 minutes. Add the white wine and reduce the liquid by half. Add the stock, bouquet garni, tomatoes, parsley, orange zest, saffron, fennel seeds, and bring to a boil. Reduce heat, add the fish, and simmer until the fish starts to flake. Remove the bouquet garni and orange zest. Skim the surface, adjust seasonings, and serve immediately.

For this soup, these fish work best: cod, sea-bream, eel, haddock, hake, mackerel, monkfish, perch, red snapper, or white fish. Remember the total calories will vary depending on the fish selected.

This soup can be refrigerated for 2 days, and can be frozen up to 1 month.

> **Per Serving:** 447 Cal (16% from Fat, 74% from Protein, 10% from Carb); 76 g Protein; 7 g Tot Fat; 2 g Sat Fat; 2 g Mono Fat; 10 g Carb; 2 g Fiber; 3 g Sugar; 215 mg Calcium; 2 mg Iron; 1017 mg Sodium; 126 mg Cholesterol

White Beans and Chard Soup

Yield: 4 servings

    2 teaspoons olive oil
    6 ounces onions, chopped (about 1 medium onion)
    4 ounces carrots, chopped (about 1 small carrot)
    4 ounces celery, chopped (about 2 celery stalks)
    4 ounces red bell peppers; seeded, ribs removed and chopped (about 1 small bell pepper)
    4 ounces yellow bell peppers; seeded, ribs removed and chopped (about 1 small bell pepper)
    1 chard head, chopped
    4 cups chicken or vegetable stock (low-fat and low-sodium)
   12 ounces organic can cooked white beans
    2 tablespoons freshly minced Italian herbs
    Salt and pepper to taste

Heat the oil in a large pan over medium heat. Add the onions and sauté until slightly browned. Add the bell peppers and cook for 2 minutes. Add the chard and sauté until the chard is wilted. Add stock, beans, and herbs. Bring to a boil, adjust seasoning, and serve immediately.

Per Serving: 243 Cal (17% from Fat, 16% from Protein, 67% from Carb); 10 g Protein; 5 g Tot Fat; 1 g Sat Fat; 3 g Mono Fat; 43 g Carb; 8 g Fiber; 9 g Sugar; 154 mg Calcium; 6 mg Iron; 898 mg Sodium; 0 mg Cholesterol

Vegetable Soup

Yield: 4 servings

    2 teaspoons olive oil
    8 ounces onions, diced (about 1 large onion)
    6 ounces carrots, diced (about 1 medium carrot)
    4 ounces celery stalks, diced (about 2 celery stalks)
    6 ounces turnips, diced (about 1 medium turnip)
    6 ounces red bell-peppers, diced (about 1 medium red bell pepper)
    2 garlic cloves, minced
    6 cups chicken or vegetable stock
    1 bouquet garni
    6 ounces fresh tomatoes peeled, seeded, and diced (about 1 large tomato)
    3 ounces frozen peas
    2 tablespoons fresh parsley, minced
    Salt and pepper to taste

Make a small X incision on the top and bottom of the tomato. Blanch the tomato for 15 to 20 seconds. Place in ice-cold water to stop the cooking process. Peel, seed, and chop the tomato.

Heat the oil in a large pan over high heat. Add the onions and sauté until translucent. Add the carrots, celery stalks, bell peppers, and sauté rapidly. Add the turnips, garlic, stock, bouquet garni, and bring to a boil over high heat. Reduce heat and simmer until barely tender. Add the peas, tomatoes, and simmer for a minute. Finish with the parsley and adjust seasonings.

Option: Add whole wheat pasta, brown rice, or quinoa. You can also add chicken, turkey, venison, or buffalo meat.

Per Serving: 249 Cal (20% from Fat, 11% from Protein, 69% from Carb); 7 g Protein; 6 g Tot Fat; 1 g Sat Fat; 3 g Mono Fat; 45 g Carb; 8 g Fiber; 15 g Sugar; 115 mg Calcium; 3 mg Iron; 1312 mg Sodium; 0 mg Cholesterol

Turkey Chili

Yield: 4 servings

1   teaspoon canola oil
8   ounces onions, diced (about 1 large onion)
6   ounces yellow bell pepper; seeded, ribs removed, and diced (about 1 medium yellow bell pepper)
2   garlic cloves, minced
1   pound ground turkey meat
1   can (15 ounces) diced tomatoes
2   ounces tomato paste

1 ¼ cup beef stock
12 ounces cooked kidney beans or pinto beans
1   teaspoon thyme
1   teaspoon oregano
2   teaspoons cumin
2   tablespoons chili powder
1/4 teaspoon cayenne pepper
Salt to taste

Heat the oil in a deep pan over high heat. Add the meat and brown slightly. Remove the excess fat rendered by the meat. Add the onion, pepper, garlic, and mix well. Stir in the tomatoes, tomato paste, stock, herbs, and spices. Bring to a boil and reduce heat. Simmer uncovered for 50 minutes to an hour. Stir occasionally. Add the beans and bring to a simmer. Adjust seasonings and serve immediately.

Per Serving: 352 Cal (15% from Fat, 41% from Protein, 44% from Carb); 37 g Protein; 6 g Tot Fat; 1 g Sat Fat; 2 g Mono Fat; 40 g Carb; 11 g Fiber; 9 g Sugar; 113 mg Calcium; 7 mg Iron; 642 mg Sodium; 74 mg Cholesterol

Side Dishes/ Desserts

Oftentimes, proteins are the focus of meals. However, you must not forget about the importance of side dishes and snacks. For one thing, their nutritional value can help complete a day's minimum requirements for vitamin and mineral intake. Once more, carefully chosen snacks and side dishes keep us from becoming bored with food. This is key, for it is often boredom that leads us to binge on poor food choices.

Side dishes should emphasize plenty of vegetables and include an appropriate amount of complex carbohydrates based on your daily activities.

Always keep the fat content low in your snacks and side dishes. Snacks should not be limited to food bars, but should instead feature fresh food sources, such as fruits, vegetables, or nuts. Good high protein snack choices also include cottage cheese and yogurt.

In the following section, you will find low-fat snack and side dish recipes that also feature the right balance of proteins and carbohydrates. This aids absorption of the nutrients and helps keep your metabolism up.

At the end of this section, you will also find several dessert options. No need to worry—although recipes like Chocolate and Hazelnut Pudding and Almond Chocolate Squares are certainly delicious, these are not your traditional, high-fat desserts. Instead, these healthy alternatives give you the freedom to treat yourself while still fulfilling the requirements for a healthy, fat-burning, and muscle-building diet.

Roasted Sweet Potatoes with Ginger

Yield: 2 servings

2 small sweet potatoes (about 5 ounces each)
2 teaspoons grapeseed oil
Ground ginger to taste
Ground cinnamon to taste
Salt and pepper to taste

Wash and pat dry the sweet potatoes. Prick the potatoes with a fork and microwave on high for 4 to 5 minutes. Transfer each potato to aluminum foil, close, and let stand for another 3 to 4 minutes.
   Preheat the broiler. Remove potatoes from foil, cut in half, and spread the grapeseed oil over the potato flesh. Sprinkle ginger, cinnamon, and season to taste. Broil until golden brown and serve immediately.

Per Serving (5 ounces sweet potato): 151 Cal (27% from Fat, 6% from Protein, 67% from Carb); 2 g Protein; 5 g Tot Fat; 0 g Sat Fat; 1 g Mono Fat; 26 g Carb; 4 g Fiber; 6 g Sugar; 44 mg Calcium; 1 mg Iron; 19 mg Sodium; 0 mg Cholesterol

Dandelion with Garlic

Yield: 2 servings

1 pound dandelion
2 teaspoons olive oil
1 garlic clove, minced
2 tablespoons vegetable broth (low-fat and low-sodium)
Salt and pepper to taste

Clean thoroughly the dandelion and dry with a salad spinner. Chop the dandelion. Heat the oil and garlic in a saucepan over medium heat. Add the dandelion and cook for 5 minutes mixing occasionally. Add the broth and season to taste. Continue to cook for another 5 minutes or until tender. Serve immediately.

Per Serving: 152 Cal (32% from Fat, 15% from Protein, 53% from Carb); 7 g Protein; 6 g Tot Fat; 1 g Sat Fat; 3 g Mono Fat; 23 g Carb; 8 g Fiber; 9 g Sugar; 437 mg Calcium; 7 mg Iron; 174 mg Sodium; 0 mg Cholesterol

Penne with Arugula and Tomatoes

Yield: 2 servings

1/2 cup to 2/3 cup whole wheat penne
2 teaspoons olive oil
6 ounces mushrooms, sliced
6 ounces orange bell peppers; seeded, ribs removed, and diced
2 garlic cloves, minced
2 large tomatoes, diced (about 12 ounces)

1/2 cup vegetable broth (low-fat and low-sodium)
2 bunches arugula, chopped
2 teaspoons parmesan cheese
2 tablespoons freshly minced basil
Salt and pepper to taste

Cook the pasta according to package directions.
Heat the oil in a nonstick pan over high heat. Add the mushrooms, garlic, and cook until golden brown. Add the bell pepper, tomatoes, and sauté quickly. Add the stock and bring to boil. Reduce heat and continue to simmer for 3 minutes. Add the arugula and cook until wilted. Mix in the cooked pasta, basil, and season to taste. Sprinkle the cheese just before serving.

Per Serving (1/2 cup cooked penne): 257 Cal (23% from Fat, 14% from Protein, 63% from Carb); 9 g Protein; 7 g Tot Fat; 1 g Sat Fat; 4 g Mono Fat; 44 g Carb; 7 g Fiber; 8 g Sugar; 88 mg Calcium; 2 mg Iron; 252 mg Sodium; 2 mg Cholesterol
Per Serving (3/4 cup cooked penne): 288 Cal (21% from Fat, 13% from Protein, 66% from Carb); 10 g Protein; 7 g Tot Fat; 1 g Sat Fat; 4 g Mono Fat; 51 g Carb; 8 g Fiber; 8 g Sugar; 89 mg Calcium; 2 mg Iron; 252 mg Sodium; 2 mg Cholesterol

Asian Noodles with Peanuts

Yield: 2 servings

1 teaspoon canola oil
1 garlic clove, minced
2 teaspoons ginger, minced
2 teaspoons low-sodium soy sauce
2 teaspoons rice vinegar
3 to 4 ounces Asian noodles
6 ounces carrots, sliced diagonally (about 1 large carrot)

4 green onions, sliced diagonally
2 tablespoons peanuts
2 tablespoons Thai basil
1 tablespoon sesame oil
Pepper to taste
Dry red pepper flakes to taste

Cook the noodles according to package instructions.
Heat the canola oil in a wok over medium heat. Add garlic, ginger, carrots and sauté 1 minute. Add green onions and sauté briefly. Add the soy sauce, rice vinegar, peanuts, basil, red pepper flakes, and bring to a boil. Add the noodles and toss to blend. Finish by adding the sesame oil, pepper to taste, and serve immediately.

Per Serving (3 ounces uncooked noodles): 315 Cal (30% from Fat, 10% from Protein, 60% from Carb); 8 g Protein; 11 g Tot Fat; 1 g Sat Fat; 5 g Mono Fat; 48 g Carb; 6 g Fiber; 5 g Sugar; 92 mg Calcium; 2 mg Iron; 1182 mg Sodium; 0 mg Cholesterol
Per Serving (4 ounces uncooked noodles): 366 Cal (26% from Fat, 10% from Protein, 64% from Carb); 10 g Protein; 11 g Tot Fat; 1 g Sat Fat; 5 g Mono Fat; 59 g Carb; 7 g Fiber; 5 g Sugar; 95 mg Calcium; 2 mg Iron; 1443 mg Sodium; 0 mg Cholesterol

Eggplant Mediterranean

Yield: 2 servings

1   pound eggplant, both ends trimmed
    (about 2 small eggplants)
2   tablespoons olive oil
1   teaspoon cumin
1   tablespoon paprika
1   tablespoon ground ginger
1   tablespoon garlic powder

1   teaspoon coriander
1/2 teaspoon cayenne pepper
1/4 teaspoon ground thyme
1/4 teaspoon ground oregano
Salt

Cut eggplant slices lengthwise and arrange on a baking sheet.
    Mix all the spices together. On both sides of the eggplant, brush olive oil, season with salt, and sprinkle the prepared spices.

Preheat the broiler or barbecue. Broil or grill until golden brown, about 2 minutes per side.

If ground thyme and oregano are difficult to find, use regular ones and mince as small as possible.

Per Serving: 199 Cal (61% from Fat, 6% from Protein, 33% from Carb); 3 g Protein; 15 g Tot Fat; 2 g Sat Fat; 10 g Mono Fat; 18 g Carb; 9 g Fiber; 6 g Sugar; 52 mg Calcium; 3 mg Iron; 10 mg Sodium; 0 mg Cholesterol

Green Beans with Almonds

Yield: 2 servings

2   cups green beans, trimmed
2   tablespoons sliced almonds
2   teaspoons grapeseed oil
1   garlic clove, minced
Salt and pepper to taste

Place the green beans in a pan and cover with water. Add 1 teaspoon of salt and bring to a boil over high heat.
    Reduce heat and simmer until crisp, about 5 to 6 minutes. Drain and set aside. Briefly heat the oil with the garlic, almonds, and add the green beans. Mix well with the beans, season to taste, and serve immediately.

Per Serving: 130 Cal (49% from Fat, 12% from Protein, 39% from Carb); 4 g Protein; 8 g Tot Fat; 1 g Sat Fat; 3 g Mono Fat; 14 g Carb; 5 g Fiber; 2 g Sugar; 81 mg Calcium; 2 mg Iron; 9 mg Sodium; 0 mg Cholesterol

Sugar Snap Peas with Garlic

Yield: 2 servings

1 tablespoon olive oil
2 cups sugar snap peas
4 garlic cloves, sliced
1 lemon
Salt and pepper to taste

Remove strings along both lengths of the sugar snap peas. Heat a wok with the olive oil over medium heat. Add the garlic and sauté quickly. Add the sugar snap peas and sauté until tender and crisp. Sprinkle a little lemon juice, season to taste and serve immediately.

Per Serving: 230 Cal (27% from Fat, 16% from Protein, 57% from Carb); 10 g Protein; 8 g Tot Fat; 1 g Sat Fat; 5 g Mono Fat; 36 g Carb; 11 g Fiber; 9 g Sugar; 121 mg Calcium; 3 mg Iron; 14 mg Sodium; 0 mg Cholesterol

Brown Rice with Mushrooms

Yield: 2 servings

2 teaspoons grapeseed oil
2/5 to 5/8 cup brown rice
1 cup to 1 ¼ cup stock or water
4 ounces onions, diced
12 ounces mushrooms, diced
1 tablespoon chives, minced
Salt and pepper to taste

Rinse the rice well and drain. Heat 1 teaspoon oil in a pan over high heat. Add the rice and sauté for a minute. Add the stock or water and bring to a boil. Cover, reduce heat, and cook until tender or about 45 minutes. Time may vary, for best results refer to package instructions.

Heat the remaining oil in a pan over high heat. Add the onion and slightly brown. Add the mushrooms and sauté until golden brown. Add the chives and season to taste. Transfer to the rice and serve immediately.

Per Serving (1/2 cup cooked brown rice): 140 Cal (22% from Fat, 14% from Protein, 64% from Carb); 5 g Protein; 4 g Tot Fat; 0 g Sat Fat; 1 g Mono Fat; 23 g Carb; 2 g Fiber; 4 g Sugar; 20 mg Calcium; 1 mg Iron; 207 mg Sodium; 1 mg Cholesterol
Per Serving (3/4 cup cooked brown rice): 184 Cal (19% from Fat, 13% from Protein, 68% from Carb); 6 g Protein; 4 g Tot Fat; 1 g Sat Fat; 1 g Mono Fat; 32 g Carb; 3 g Fiber; 4 g Sugar; 25 mg Calcium; 1 mg Iron; 259 mg Sodium; 1 mg Cholesterol

Vegetables with Tapenade

Yield: 2 servings

1 ½ ounces black olives, pitted
2   anchovy fillets, rinsed and pat dry
1 ½ teaspoon capers
1/2 small garlic clove
1   tablespoon olive oil
Lemon juice to taste
Pepper to taste
Vegetables such as carrots,
    bell peppers, cherry tomatoes,
    and mushrooms

In a food processor purée the olives, anchovies, capers, and garlic. Add pepper to taste. Slowly add the olive oil until you obtain a smooth paste. Add lemon juice to taste.

Per Serving: 104 Cal (79% from Fat, 7% from Protein, 14% from Carb); 2 g Protein; 9 g Tot Fat; 1 g Sat Fat; 7 g Mono Fat; 4 g Carb; 1 g Fiber; 0 g Sugar; 42 mg Calcium; 1 mg Iron; 397 mg Sodium; 3 mg Cholesterol (without vegetables)

Half Red Bell Pepper Stuffed with Tuna

Yield: 2 servings

6 to 8 ounces can tuna
1/2 teaspoon paprika
2   teaspoons fine herbs
1/2 teaspoon garlic powder
1   ounce onion, diced small
    (about 1/4 small onion)
1 ½ ozs carrot, diced (about half a carrot)

1   ounce celery stalk, diced small
    (about 1 celery stalk)
2   tablespoons low-fat canola mayonnaise
6   ounces red bell pepper, cut in half, seeded
    and ribs removed
Salt and pepper to taste

Mix the tuna, paprika, fine herbs, onions, carrots, celery, and mayonnaise in a bowl. Season to taste and refrigerate for 30 minutes.
Equally divide the tuna mixture between the two halves and serve immediately.

Per Serving (3 ounces tuna): 167 Cal (21% from Fat, 51% from Protein, 29% from Carb); 21 g Protein; 4 g Tot Fat; 1 g Sat Fat; 1 g Mono Fat; 12 g Carb; 3 g Fiber; 6 g Sugar; 38 mg Calcium; 1 mg Iron; 75 mg Sodium; 42 mg Cholesterol
Per Serving (4 ounces tuna): 198 Cal (19% from Fat, 57% from Protein, 24% from Carb); 28 g Protein; 4 g Tot Fat; 1 g Sat Fat; 1 g Mono Fat; 12 g Carb; 3 g Fiber; 6 g Sugar; 43 mg Calcium; 1 mg Iron; 86 mg Sodium; 54 mg Cholesterol

Radishes with Hazelnut Cream Cheese

Yield: 1 serving

10 radishes
1 tablespoon low-fat sour cream
1 teaspoon low-fat milk
1 tablespoon hazelnuts
Pinch of salt
Pinch of pepper

Crush and mince the hazelnuts with a chef knife. Mix the sour cream with the yogurt in a bowl. Add the minced hazelnuts, salt, and pepper. Serve immediately with the radishes.

Variation: Mix in a little horseradish or fine herbs.

Per Serving: 79 Cal (63% from Fat, 12% from Protein, 24% from Carb); 3 g Protein; 6 g Tot Fat; 1 g Sat Fat; 4 g Mono Fat; 5 g Carb; 2 g Fiber; 3 g Sugar; 45 mg Calcium; 1 mg Iron; 58 mg Sodium; 4 mg Cholesterol

Cottage Cheese, Raisins, and Walnuts

Yield: 1 serving

1/3 cup 2% cottage cheese, cold
1 tablespoon chopped walnuts
2 teaspoons raisins
Cinnamon to taste

Mix cottage cheese, walnut, and raisins. Sprinkle cinnamon to taste and serve immediately.

Per Serving: 136 Cal (40% from Fat, 33% from Protein, 26% from Carb); 12 g Protein; 6 g Tot Fat; 1 g Sat Fat; 1 g Mono Fat; 9 g Carb; 1 g Fiber; 5 g Sugar; 63 mg Calcium; 0 mg Iron; 307 mg Sodium; 6 mg Cholesterol

Apple and Almond Butter

Yield: 1 serving

1 small apple (about 4 ounces)
1 tablespoon almond butter

Cut the apple in half, remove core, and slice. Equally spread the almond butter among the slices.

Per Serving: 153 Cal (51% from Fat, 6% from Protein, 43% from Carb); 3 g Protein; 9 g Tot Fat; 1 g Sat Fat; 6 g Mono Fat; 18 g Carb; 2 g Fiber; 11 g Sugar; 48 mg Calcium; 1 mg Iron; 2 mg Sodium; 0 mg Cholesterol

Chocolate Pudding

Yield: 3 servings

1¼ cup low-fat milk
3   extra large egg yolks
4   tablespoons sugar
2   tablespoons cornstarch
1   teaspoon orange extract
1   teaspoon orange zest
3   tablespoons Dutch cocoa powder

Bring the milk to a boil in a saucepan. Whisk the egg yolks, sugar, cocoa, orange zest, and cornstarch in a bowl until smooth. Temper the egg mixture with a little hot milk, stirring with a whisk. Transfer the mixture to the remaining hot milk, whisking rapidly and constantly. Heat over medium heat and bring to a boil, whisking the bottom and sides of the pan to avoid scorching. The mixture will thicken in about a minute. Continue to cook and whisk until a nice shine appears, about another minute. Mix in the orange extract and divide among 3 ramekins. Place a plastic wrap over the surface of each pudding and allow cooling a bit at room temperature. Refrigerate for 2 hours and serve cold.

Per Serving: 210 Cal (32% from Fat, 15% from Protein, 53% from Carb); 9 g Protein; 8 g Tot Fat; 4 g Sat Fat; 3 g Mono Fat; 31 g Carb; 5 g Fiber; 18 g Sugar; 159 mg Calcium; 2 mg Iron; 53 mg Sodium; 213 mg Cholesterol

Pomegranate and Strawberry Parfait

Yield: 2 servings

1½ cup strawberries
2   ounces pure Acai, no sugar added
    (1 Sambazon smoothie pack)
1   teaspoon vanilla extract
1   cup low-fat yogurt
2   tablespoons pomegranate seeds

Defrost Acai.
    Mix the strawberries with vanilla extract and Acai. Marinade for 30 minutes. Spoon half the fruit mixture into four serving parfait glasses. Top with yogurt and finish with the berries. Sprinkle the pomegranate seeds and serve immediately.

Option: Add Protein Powder and/or ground flaxseeds. You may substitute cottage cheese for yogurt.

Per Serving: 138 Cal (16% from Fat, 22% from Protein, 62% from Carb); 7 g Protein; 2 g Tot Fat; 1 g Sat Fat; 1 g Mono Fat; 21 g Carb; 3 g Fiber; 16 g Sugar; 249 mg Calcium; 1 mg Iron; 87 mg Sodium; 7 mg Cholesterol

Fruit with Chocolate Sauce

Yield: 2 servings

1/2 cup strawberries
1/2 cup orange slices
1/2 cup peach slices
1   kiwi, sliced
1 ½ ounce semi-sweet chocolate, shredded
1 ½ tablespoon water

Equally divide the fruits among two plates.
Melt the chocolate with water over low heat in a double boiler. Whisk until smooth. If necessary, add a little more water. Drizzle the hot chocolate sauce over the fruits and serve immediately.

Per Serving: 179 Cal (31% from Fat, 5% from Protein, 64% from Carb); 2 g Protein; 7 g Tot Fat; 4 g Sat Fat; 2 g Mono Fat; 32 g Carb; 5 g Fiber; 25 g Sugar; 49 mg Calcium; 1 mg Iron; 5 mg Sodium; 0 mg Cholesterol

Pear and Apple Minestrone

Yield: 2 servings

5   ounces apples, brunoise (about 1 apple)
5   ounces pears, brunoise (about 1 pear)
3/4 cup jasmine green tea (or your favorite)
1 ½ teaspoon honey
1/2 teaspoon pumpkin pie spices
1   small ginger root, minced
1/2 teaspoon lemon zest
1/2 teaspoon grapeseed oil

Heat the oil in a deep saucepan over high heat. Add the apples and sauté for two minutes. Add the pears, spices, ginger, lemon zest, and sauté another minute. Add the green tea and bring to a boil. Remove from heat and transfer to a serving bowl. Cool at room temperature. Refrigerate for an hour (or best overnight) to allow flavors to develop. Serve cold.

Per Serving: 105 Cal (10% from Fat, 2% from Protein, 88% from Carb); 1 g Protein; 1 g Tot Fat; 0 g Sat Fat; 0 g Mono Fat; 25 g Carb; 3 g Fiber; 18 g Sugar; 19 mg Calcium; 1 mg Iron; 2 mg Sodium; 0 mg Cholesterol

Thin Peach Tart

Yield: 8 servings

- 3 ounces almond meal
- 2 ounces oats
- 3 tablespoons grapeseed oil
- 1 tablespoon almond extract
- 2 to 3 tablespoons ice cold water
- 2 tablespoons peach preserves
- 1 pound peaches (about 4 peaches)
- Pinch salt

Preheat the oven to 475°F.
Place the oats in a blender and reduce to a flour consistency. Place the oat and almond flours in a bowl. Add salt, oil, almond extract, and mix until crumbly. Add one tablespoon water at a time and continue until the dough is smooth and sticks together as one ball. Lay the dough on wax paper and push down with your palm to flatten a bit. Roll out the dough to a round thin form. Turn over the dough to a cookie sheet. Brush 1 tablespoon preserves all over the pie dough surface.

Peel the peaches and cut in half. Core, quarter, and slice. Starting at the edge of the dough and working inward toward the center, arrange the slices in overlapping circles. Finish with another circle of peach slices in the center.

Bake for 15 to 20 minutes until golden brown and slightly darker around the edges. Heat the remaining preserves with a little water to thin out in the microwave. Remove the tart from the oven and brush with the preserves. Transfer the tart to a cooling rack.

Per Serving: 173 Cal (56% from Fat, 9% from Protein, 35% from Carb); 4 g Protein; 11 g Tot Fat; 1 g Sat Fat; 1 g Mono Fat; 16 g Carb; 3 g Fiber; 9 g Sugar; 31 mg Calcium; 0 mg Iron; 6 mg Sodium; 0 mg Cholesterol

High Fiber Salad

Yield: 8 servings

- 2 oranges, skin removed and sliced
- 1 granny smith apple, skin removed and diced
- 1 Anjou pear, skin removed and diced
- 1/2 cup grapes (combination of white and red)
- 1 cup strawberries
- 1/2 cup blueberries
- 1/2 cup raspberries
- 1/2 cup blackberries
- 1 mango, diced
- 1/2 pineapple, wedged
- Juice of 1 orange (or lime, lemon)

Place the fruits in a bowl. Add the orange juice and mix well. Refrigerate until use.

This is a great healthy fruit salad for a party. You may add fresh minced herbs such as rosemary, basil, or mint.

Per Serving: 127 Cal (3% from Fat, 4% from Protein, 93% from Carb); 2 g Protein; 0 g Tot Fat; 0 g Sat Fat; 0 g Mono Fat; 33g Carb; 5 g Fiber; 24 g Sugar; 46 mg Calcium; 0 mg Iron; 3 mg Sodium; 0 mg Cholesterol

Side Dishes / Desserts

Acai and Soy Milk Popsicle

Yield: 4 popsicles

3.5 ounces Pure Acai, no sugar added
    (Sambazon smoothie pack)
4 ounces berries
4 ounces banana (about a small banana)
4 ounces soy milk

Place all the fruits and soy milk in a blender. Purée on high speed. Divide equally among 4 popsicle molds and freeze.

Per Serving: 69 Cal (27% from Fat, 10% from Protein, 63% from Carb); 2 g Protein; 2 g Tot Fat; 0 g Sat Fat; 0 g Mono Fat; 12 g Carb; 3 g Fiber; 5 g Sugar; 10 mg Calcium; 0 mg Iron; 6 mg Sodium; 0 mg Cholesterol

---

Strawberries and Spinach Smoothie

Yield: 2 servings

2 cups strawberries
1 bunch fresh spinach
1 banana
1 tablespoon flaxseeds
Aged balsamic vinegar to taste (optional)
Ice cubs

Place strawberries, spinach, and banana into a blender. Puree and mix in the aged balsamic vinegar (optional). Serve immediately.

Option: Add Protein Powder which adds 100 calories

Per Serving: 178 Cal (13% from Fat, 15% from Protein, 72% from Carb); 8 g Protein; 3 g Tot Fat; 0 g Sat Fat; 0 g Mono Fat; 37 g Carb; 10 g Fiber; 17 g Sugar; 206 mg Calcium; 6 mg Iron; 138 mg Sodium; 0 mg Cholesterol

Flourless Walnut Cake with Chocolate Drizzles

Yield: 12 servings

10 ounces walnuts
3 eggs
3 ounces light brown sugar
2 ounces unsalted butter, melted and cooled
1/2 teaspoon vanilla extract

3 tablespoons Dutch cacao powder
5 to 6 tablespoons evaporated 2% milk
2 tablespoons honey
Pinch salt

Preheat the oven to 355 F. Grease an 8 inch diameter cake pan and place wax paper on the bottom of it. In a food processor, chop down the walnuts. You need to end up with a meal consistency but with still lots of small chopped nuts pieces in it in order to maintain the texture of the cake.

Separate the egg whites from the yolks. Beat the yolks with the sugar until it becomes a light pale color. Add the vanilla, salt, melted butter, and mix until well incorporated. Start to whip the egg whites, adding a teaspoon of sugar half way through. Once the egg whites are firm, fold a third of it into the prepared mixture. Add remaining egg whites while folding carefully not to break them. Transfer to the cake pan and bake for 40 minutes or until a cake pick inserted in the center comes out dry. Be aware that the cake will not rise much—that is normal. Cool over a rack before unmolding. Remove wax paper and cut into 12 slices.

Mix the cacao and evaporated milk. Add the honey and warm up in the microwave for 15 to 20 seconds. Mix again before use. Plate each cake slice, drizzle 1 tablespoon chocolate sauce, and serve immediately.

Many twists can be given to this basic recipe. Keep in mind it will change calories.

- Melt 1 teaspoon almond butter into the chocolate sauce
- Add 1 apple, diced into the cake mixture
- Add cinnamon into the cake mixture
- Substitute the vanilla with rum or walnut liquor
- Substitute butter with grapeseed oil. Be aware it will change the cake texture and flavor.

Per Serving: 254 Cal (70% from Fat, 9% from Protein, 21% from Carb); 6 g Protein; 21 g Tot Fat; 4 g Sat Fat; 4 g Mono Fat; 14 g Carb; 2 g Fiber; 10 g Sugar; 60 mg Calcium; 1 mg Iron; 30 mg Sodium; 72 mg Cholesterol

Recipes inspired from:

THE SAINT-TROPEZ DIET
—*Apostolos Pappas, Marie-Annick Courtier*

THE PARK AVENUE DIET
—*Dr. Stuart Fisher, Marie-Annick Courtier*

THE PROFESSIONAL CHEF
—*Culinary Institute of America*

THE FLAVORS OF BON APPETIT 1998

FRENCH CLASSICS
—*Richard Grausman*